Plant-Based D

Begin

Amazing Quick and Easy Plant-Based Recipes to Boost Your Diet and Satisfy Your Taste

Sheryl Ward

Table of Contents

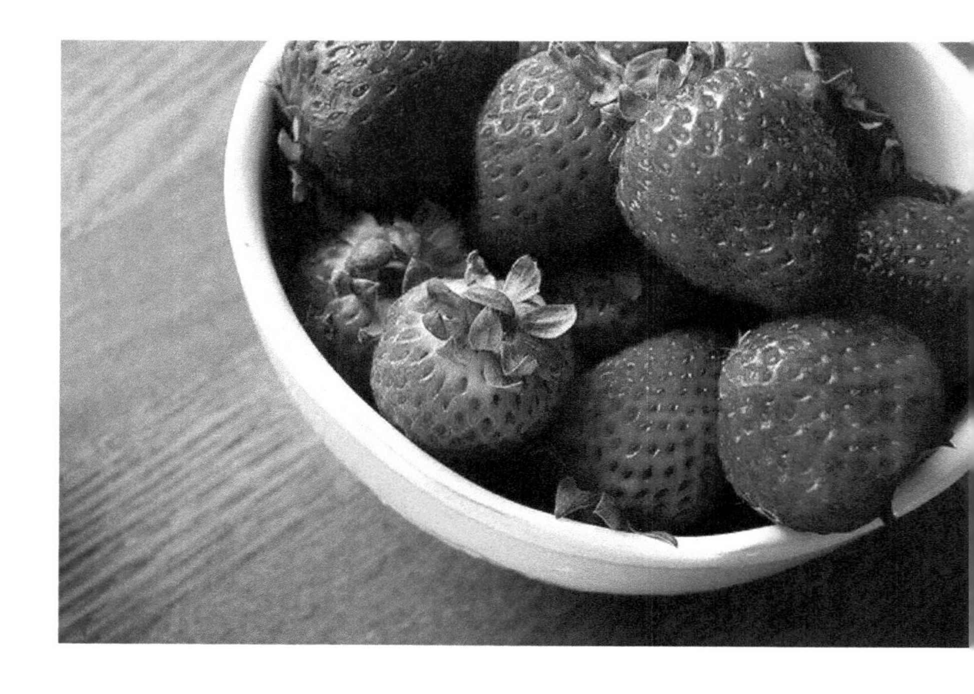

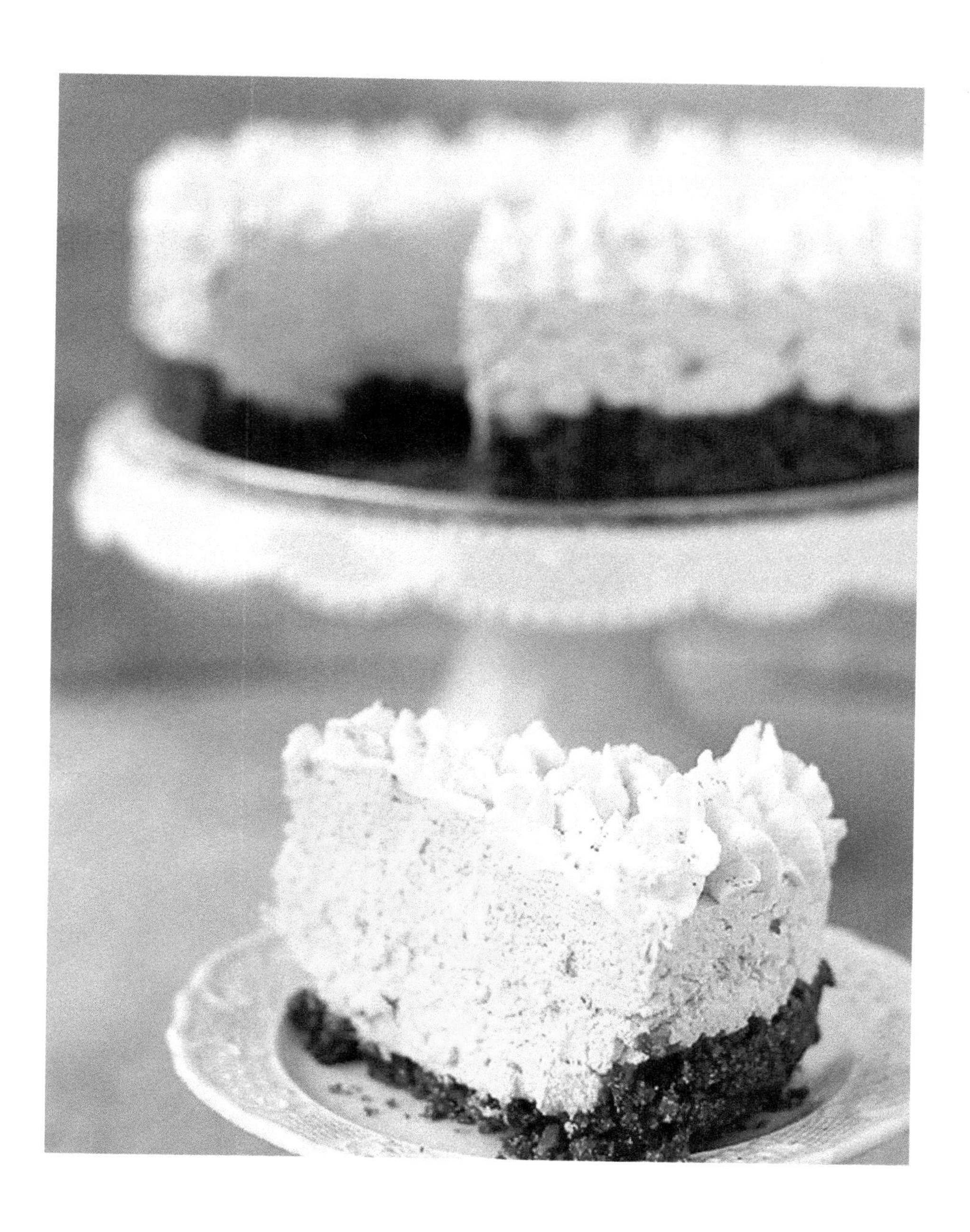

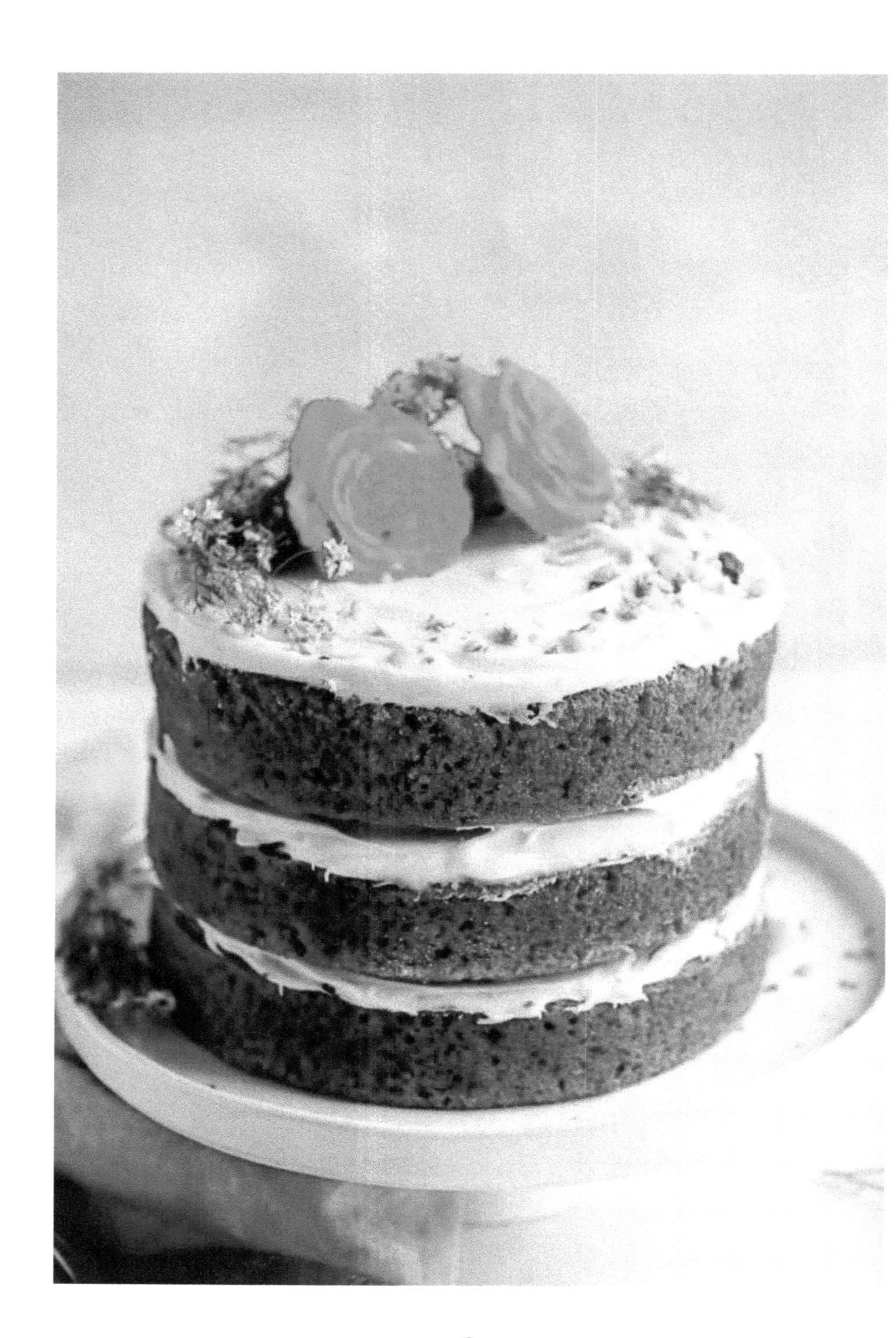

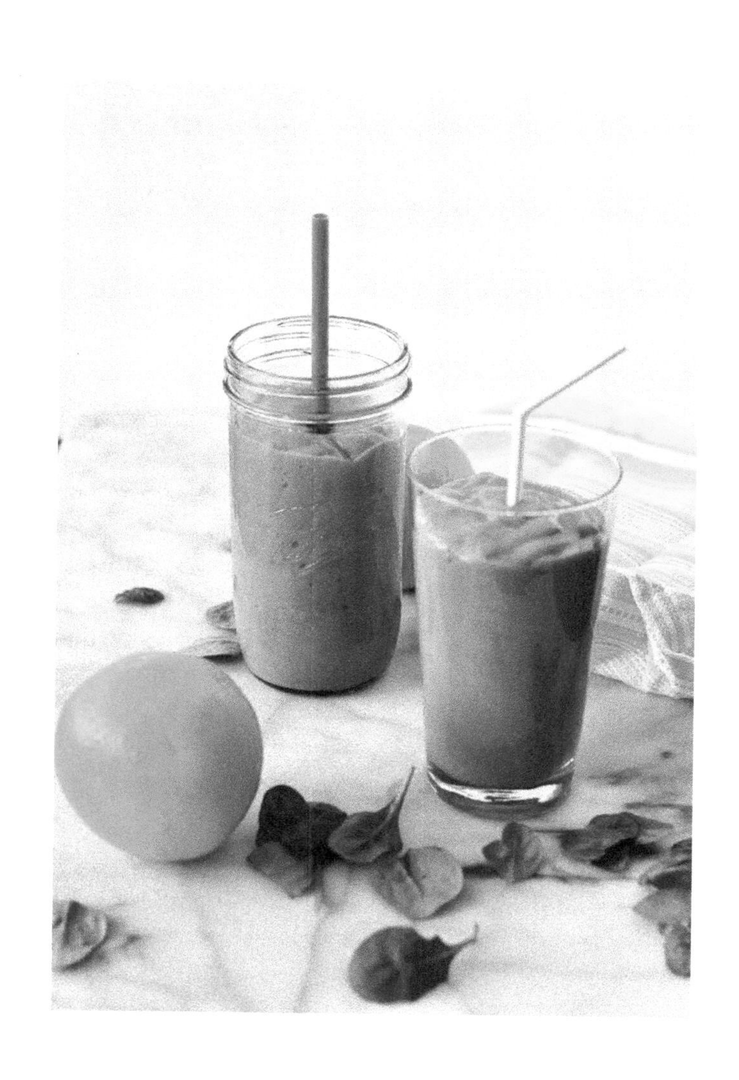

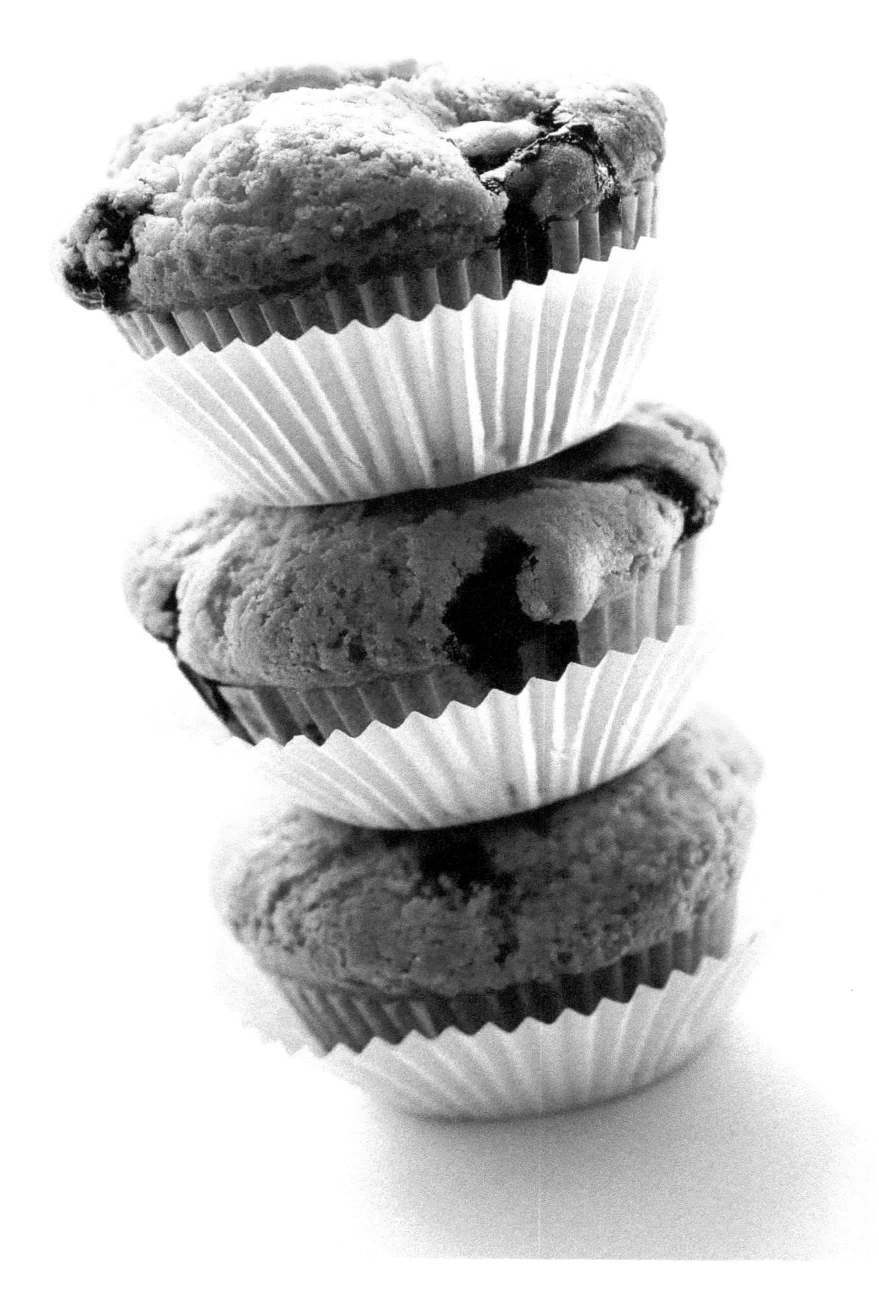

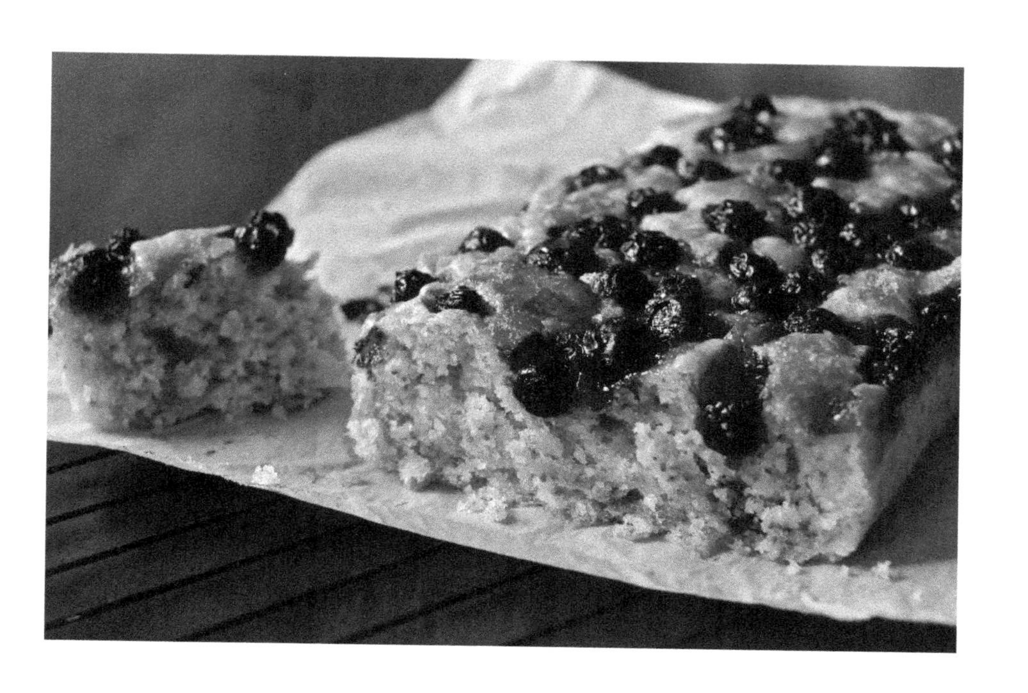

No-bake chocolate chip cookies

Preparation time: 5 minutes | Cooking time: 20 minutes | Servings: 12

Ingredients:

2 tbsp. butter 3 tbsp. milk 1 tsp vanilla extract ½ tsp salt ½ cup brown sugar 1 ½ cup oat flour ½ cup of chocolate chips

Directions: Take a large bowl, pour the melted butter and brown sugar and whisk it for a minute. After that, add milk and vanilla extract into it. Now add the oat flour, salt and stir well until a dough formed. Add the chocolate chips in the dough and fold them well. Set parchment paper in the cookie pan and set it aside. Take dough balls and turn them into cookie shape with hand. Make 12 cookies and place them into the cookie tray. Garnish the cookies with additional chocolate chips. Put them in the refrigerator for 20 minutes. Serve and store for up to 10 days.

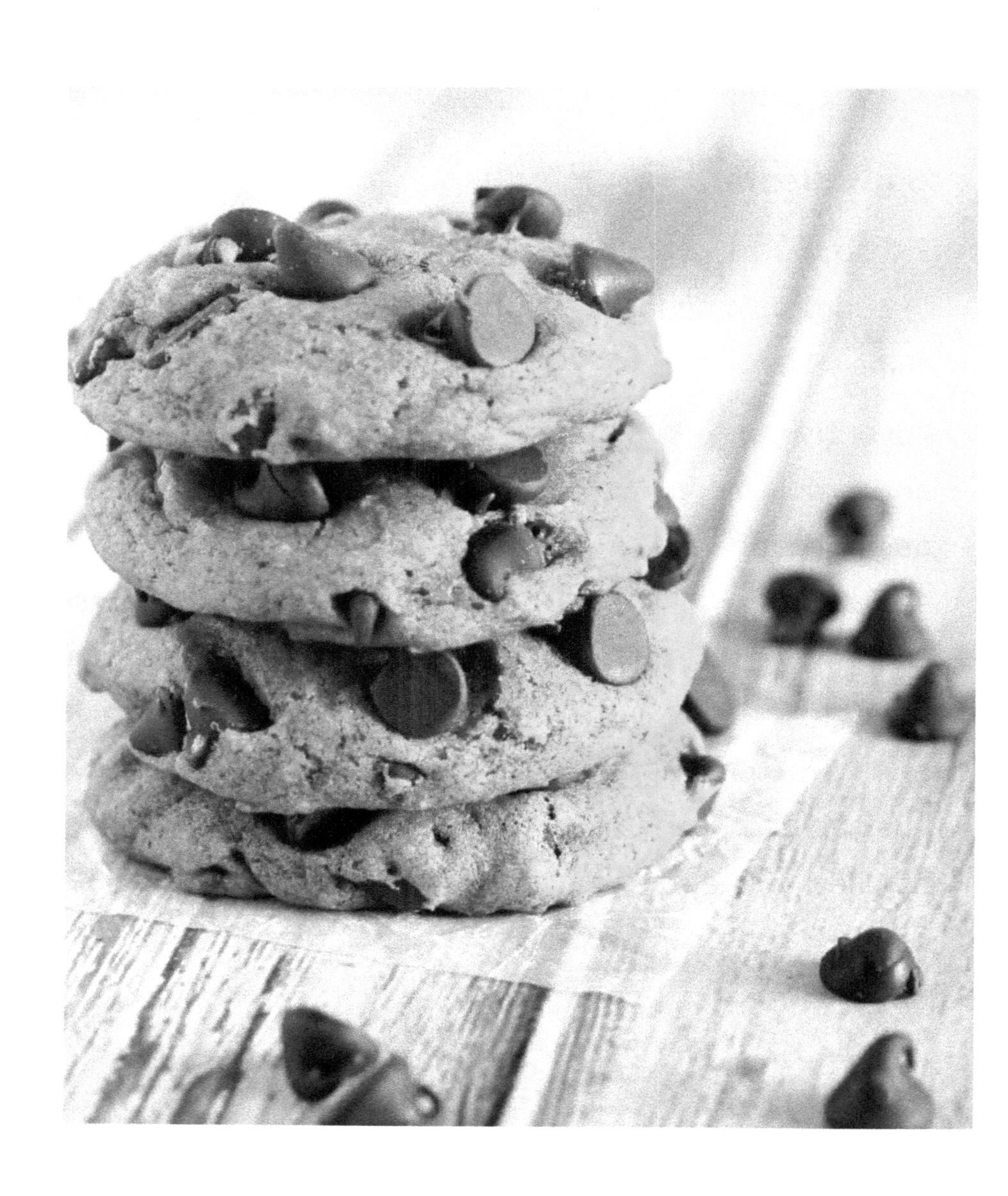

Sea salt butterscotch tart

Preparation time: 20 minutes | Cooking time: 30 minutes | Servings: 10

Ingredients:

½ cup of sugar 2 cups almond flour ¼ cup of coconut oil ½ tsp salt 1 tsp vanilla extract For filling: 2/3 cup brown sugar or coconut sugar 2/3 cup coconut cream ½ cup of coconut oil 1tsp salt Flaked sea salt 1 smith apple

Directions:

Preheat the oven at 375 degrees and set a round tart pand set aside. For crust: In a mixing bowl, add sugar, coconut oil, vanilla extract and mix until fluffy. Add the almond flour and salt in the mixture to mix the Ingredients. Pour the mixture into the tart pan and put it in the freezer for 10 minutes. After that, bake the tart into the oven for 15 minutes until it turns into brown color and crusty. For filling: Take a pan, add brown sugar, coconut cream, coconut oil and salt. Bring it to boil and cook on a medium flame for around 25 minutes. Test the filling into ice-cold water, take a folk dip into filling and then into cold water. If it remains stick without dissolving in water means your filling is ready. Pour the filling on the tart crust and spread evenly. Add the apple slice for garnish and let it cool. Serve the perfect butterscotch tart.

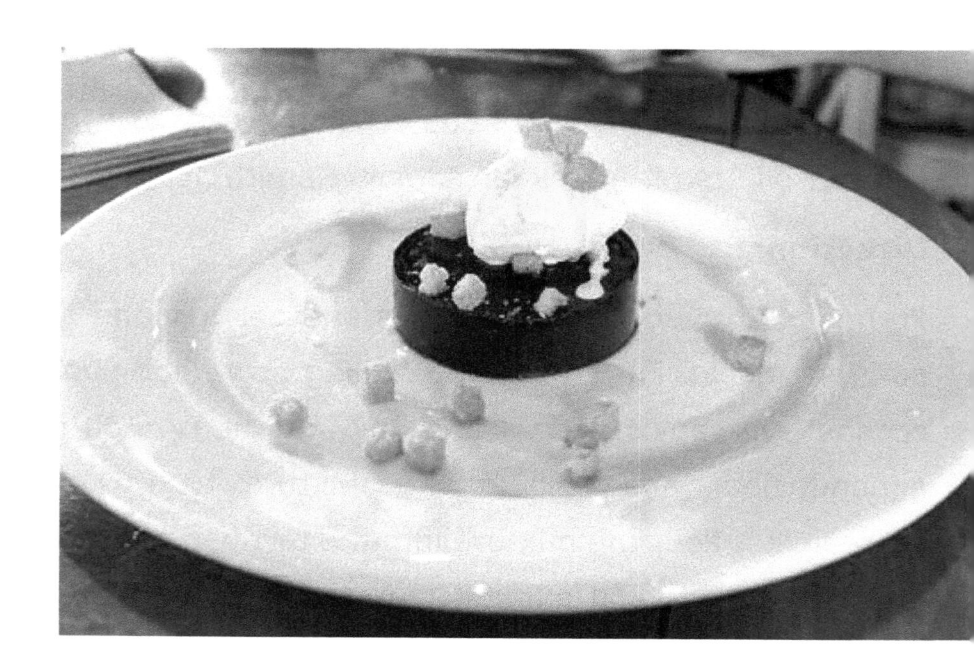

Peanut butter cream sweet potato brownies

Preparation time: 5 minutes | Cooking time: 20 minutes | Servings: 6

Ingredients:

1 cup mashed sweet potato Frosting of your choice ½ cup almond butter ¼-2/3 cup cocoa powder

Directions: Before starting, preheat the oven at 350 degrees and set a baking pan with parchment paper and place aside. Take a blender, add sweet potato, almond butter and cocoa powder and blend until well combined. After that pour the material into a baking pan and spread evenly. Bake it for 15 to 18 minutes. Let them cool and cut into equal slices. Serve the brownie slice with the frosting of your choice.

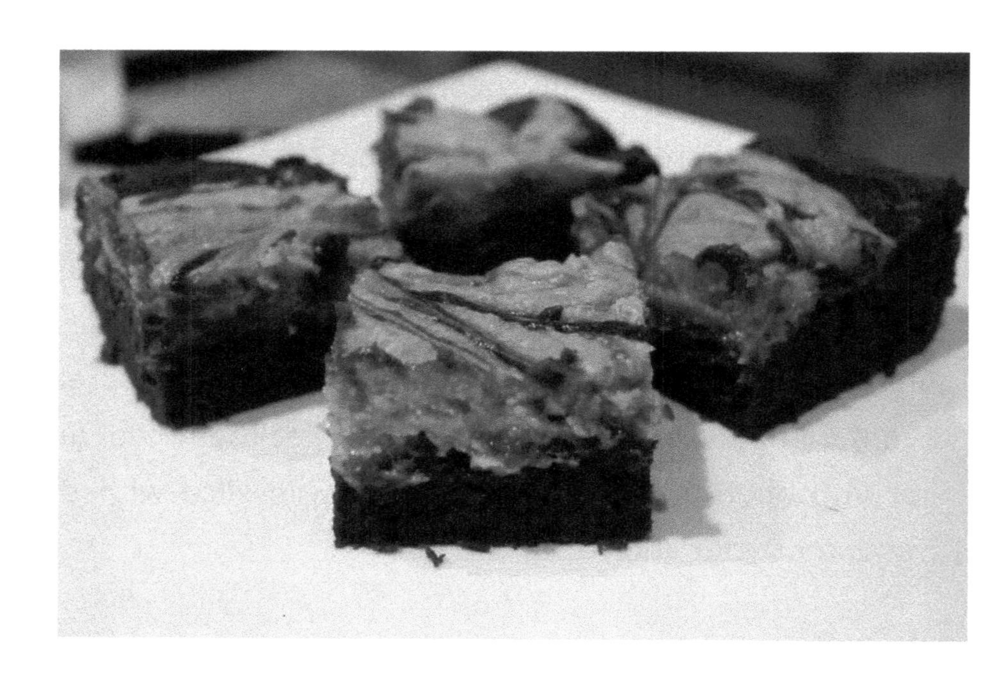

Vegan cinnamon rolls

Preparation time:1 hour 30 minutes |Cooking time:25 minutes|Servings: 10

Ingredients:

For dough: 3tbsp vegan butter 1 cup almond milk 1 pack instant yeast 1 tbsp. cane sugar ¼ tsp salt 3 cup flour

Filling: 3 tbsp. butter ¼ cup of cane sugar ½ tbsp. cinnamon Topping: 2 tbsp. butter

Directions: For the dough: take a pan, heat the butter until melted or warm in a microwave. Pour the butter in a mixing bowl and add yeast, leave it for 10 minutes. After that stir sugar and salt in it. Now add flour and keep stirring the mixture until a dough formed. Wrap the dough and set aside. Flattened the dough on the surface and makes rolls and filled with the cinnamon and sugar as per required. Put the rolls into the baking pan and brush the butter and sugar on top. Bake for 25 to 30 minutes in a preheated oven until golden brown. Let it cool and serve.

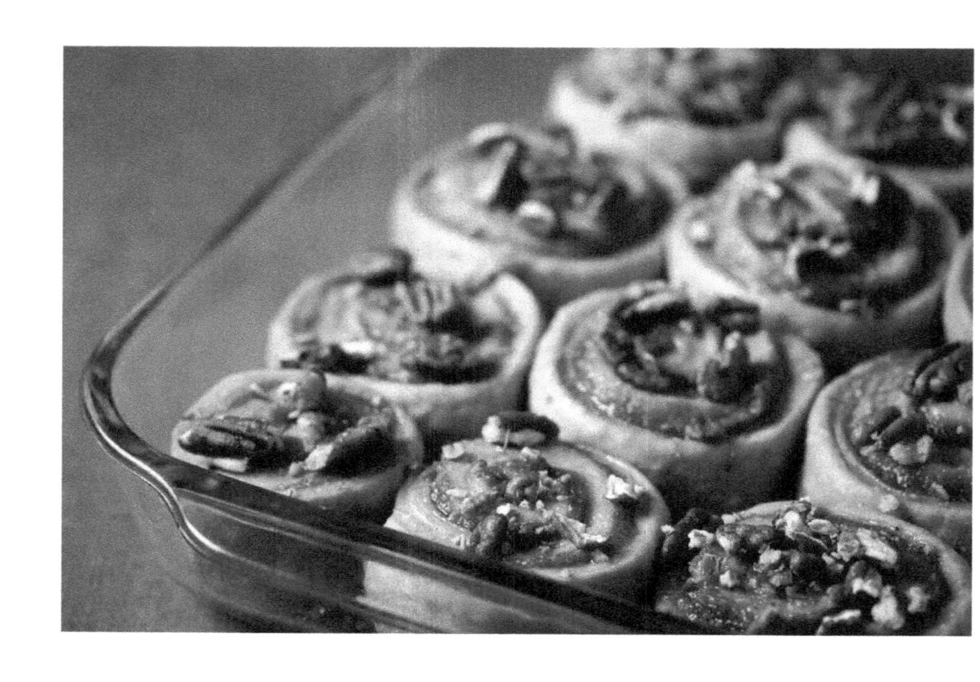

Onion Cheese Muffins

Preparation time: 20 minutes Cooking time: 20 minutes Servings: 6

Ingredients:

¼ cup Colby jack cheese, shredded ¼ cup shallots, minced 1 cup almond flour 1 egg 3 tbsp sour cream What you'll need from the store cupboard: ½ tsp salt 3 tbsp melted butter or oil

Directions

Line 6 muffin tins with 6 muffin liners. Set aside and preheat oven to 350oF. In a bowl, stir the dry and wet ingredients alternately. Mix well using a spatula until the consistency of the mixture becomes even. Scoop a spoonful of the batter to the prepared muffin tins. Bake for 20 minutes in the oven until golden brown. Serve and enjoy.

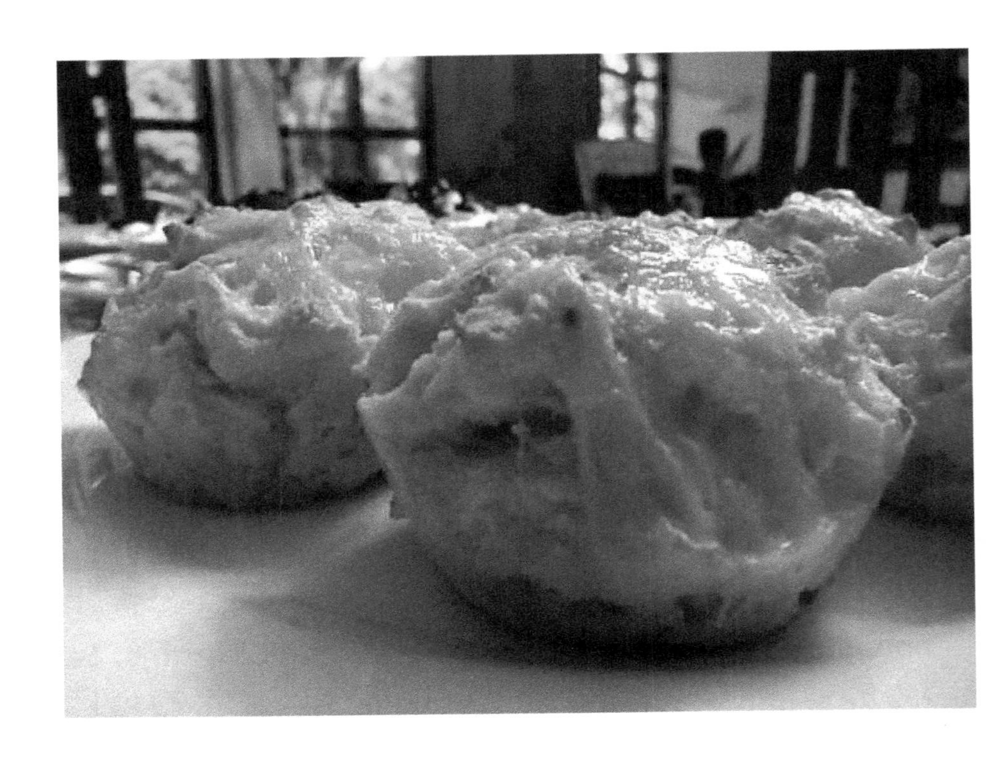

French Lover's Coconut Macaroons

Preparation time: 15 minutes Cooking time: 25 minutes 12 cookies.

Ingredients:

1/3 cup agave nectar ½ cup coconut cream 1 cup shredded coconut ½ tsp. salt 1/3 cup chocolate chips

Directions:

Begin by preheating your oven to 300 degrees Fahrenheit. Next, mix together the coconut cream, the agave, and the salt. Next, fold in the chocolate chips and the coconut. Stir well, and create cookie balls. Place the balls on a baking sheet, and bake the cookies for twenty-five minutes. Enjoy.

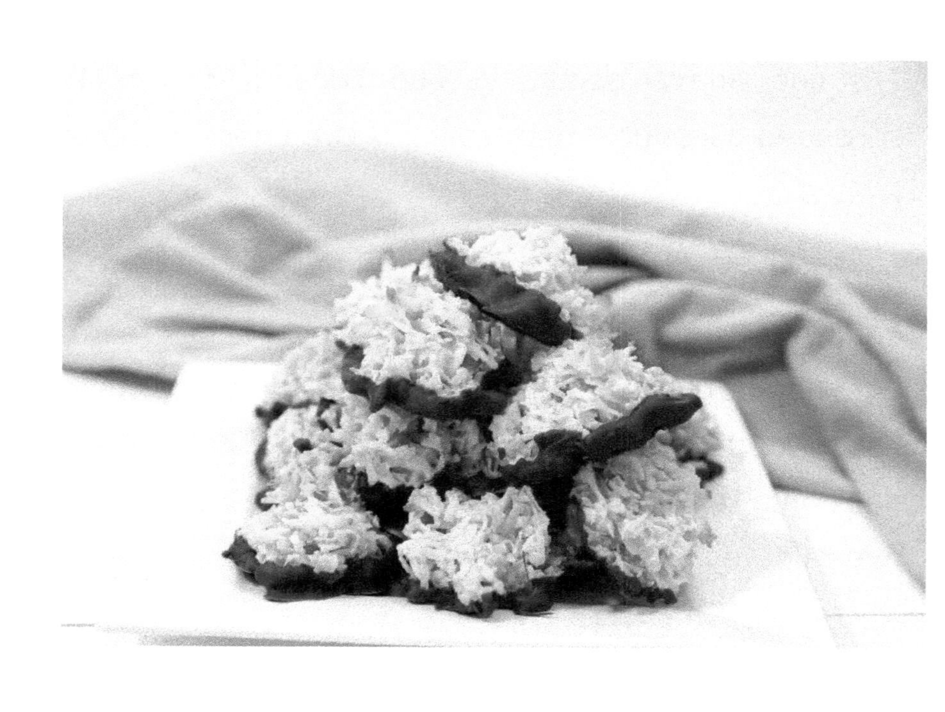

Gluten-Free Cranberry Orange Muffin

Preparation time: 15 minutes Cooking time: 15 minutes 12 muffins.

Ingredients:

2 ¼ cups oat flour 1 tsp. baking soda 1/3 cup sugar 1 tsp. salt 1 tsp. cinnamon 2 tbsp. ground flax 6 tbsp. water 2 tsp. orange zest 2 tsp. vanilla 1/3 cup almond milk ½ cup fresh-squeezed orange juice 1/3 cup melted coconut oil 1 ¼ cup craisins 1 cup diced walnuts

Directions:

Begin by preheating your oven to 350 degrees Fahrenheit. Next, bring 2 tbsp. flax seed and 6 tbsp. of water together in a small bowl. Set this bowl to the side for five minutes. Next, mix together all the dry ingredients. Afterwards, add the flax seed to the dry mixture along with the almond milk, orange juice, orange zest, and the vanilla. Administer the coconut oil at the end. Gently mix the dough and then add the cranberries and the walnuts. Pour the batter into muffin tins, and bake the muffins for twenty-five minutes. Cool the muffins prior to serving, and enjoy!

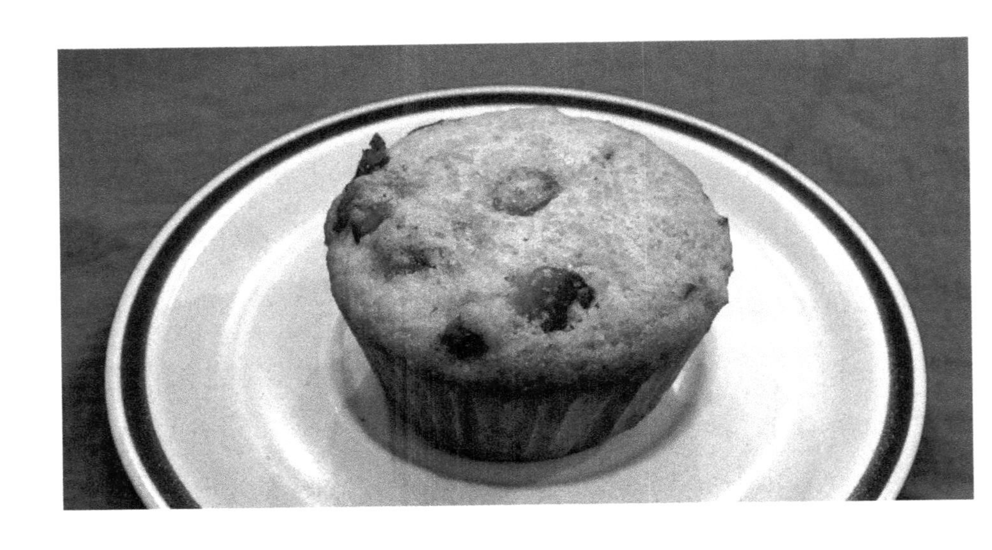

Revving Apple Parsnip Muffin

Preparation time: 15 minutes Cooking time: 45 minutes 15 muffins.

Ingredients:

1 cup walnuts 1 cup grated apple 2 cups grated parsnip 2 tsp. baking powder 2 cups all-purpose flour 1 tsp. cinnamon 1 tsp. baking soda 1 ½ tsp. ginger ½ cup raisins 1 cup melted coconut oil 1 cup almond milk ½ cup maple syrup 1 tsp. apple cider vinegar 2 tsp. vanilla

Directions: Begin by preheating your oven to 350 degrees Fahrenheit. Next, grate both your apples and your parsnips. Stir the dry ingredients together—everything except your apples and parsnips. Then, stir together the wet ingredients in a small bowl. Bring the wet ingredients into the dry ingredient bowl along with the apples and parsnips. Mix the ingredients until they're just moistened, and bake the muffins for twenty-five minutes. Allow the muffins to cool, and enjoy!

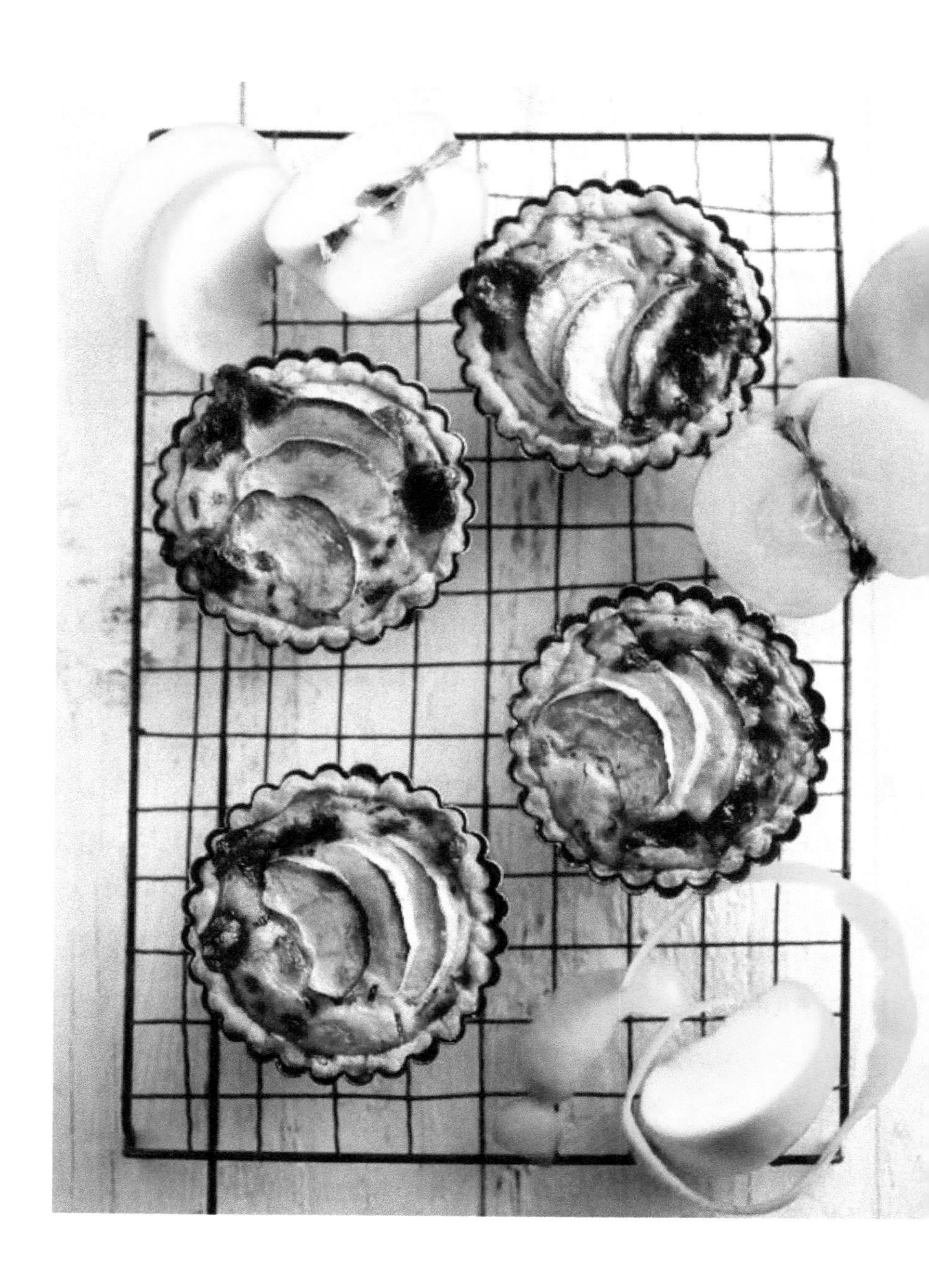

Crunchy Peanut Butter Muffins with Ginger

Preparation time: 15 minutes Cooking time: 25 minutes 10 muffins.

Ingredients:

1 cup oats 1 cup flour 2 tsp. apple cider vinegar 1 cup hot water 1/3 cup crunchy peanut butter 1/3 cup canola oil ½ cup dark brown sugar ½ cup chunky applesauce ½ tsp. baking soda 1 tsp. baking powder ½ cup candied gingers

Directions: Begin by preheating the oven to 400 degrees Fahrenheit. Next, mix together the oats, the water, and the vinegar in a large mixing bowl. Allow the mixture to sit there for about twenty minutes. Next, add the peanut butter, the oil, the sugar, and the applesauce to the mixture. Stir well. Next, sift the dry ingredients together in a different bowl. Add this mixture to the wet ingredients, next, and stir well. When you've mixed the batter, pour the batter into a muffin tin and allow the muffins to bake for fifteen minutes. After fifteen minutes, reduce the heat to 375 degrees Fahrenheit. Give the muffins another eight minutes. Next, remove the muffins and allow them to cool. Enjoy!

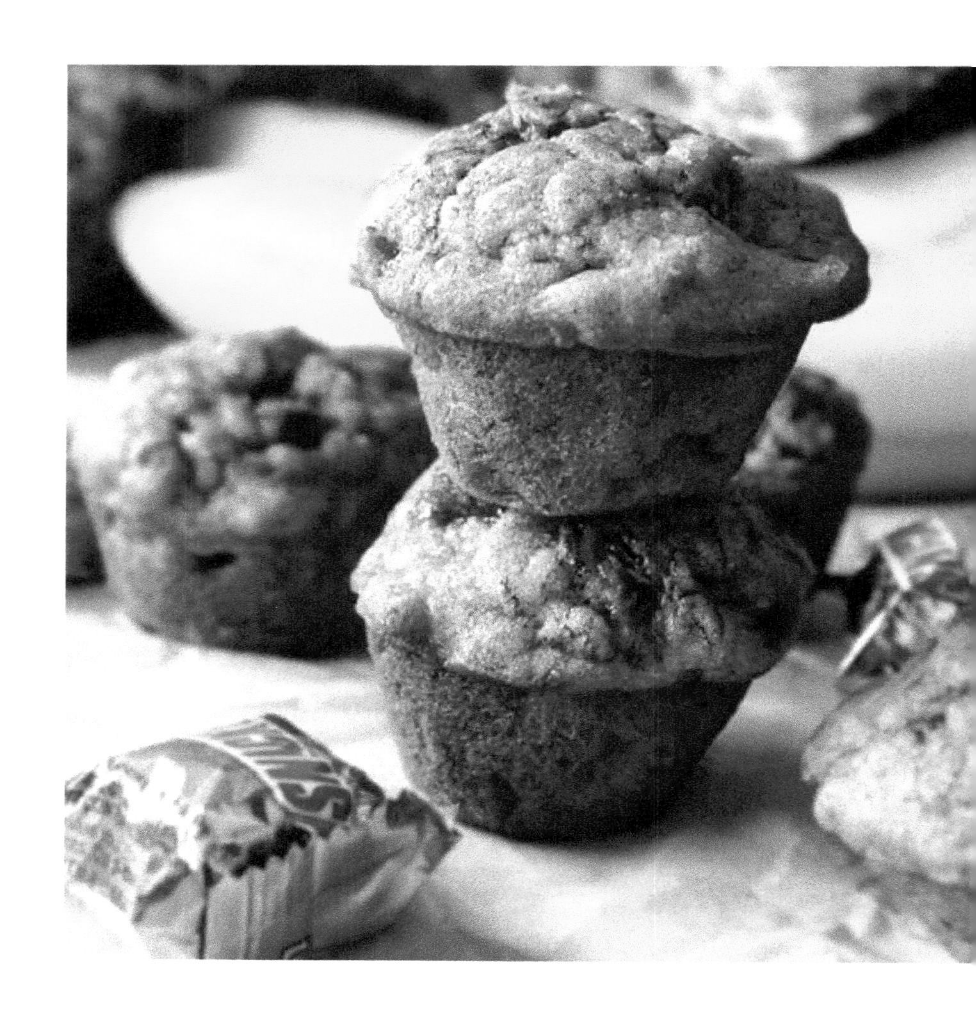

Zucchini Chocolate Crisis Bread

Preparation time: 15 minutes Cooking time: 25 minutes 1 bread loaf.

Ingredients:

1 cup sugar 2 tbsp. flax seeds 6 tbsp. water 1 cup applesauce 1/3 cup cocoa powder 2 cups all-purpose flour 2 tsp. vanilla 1 tsp. baking soda ½ tsp. baking powder 1 tbsp. cinnamon 1 tsp. salt 2 1/3 cup grated zucchini 1 cup nondairy chocolate chips

Directions:

Begin by preheating your oven to 325 degrees Fahrenheit. First, mix together the water and the flax seeds and allow the mixture to thicken to the side for five minutes. Mix all the dry ingredients together. Next, add the wet ingredients to the dry ingredients, including the flax seeds. Next, add the chocolate chips and the zucchini. Stir well, and spread the batter out into your bread loaf pan. Bake the creation for thirty minutes. Afterward it cools, enjoy!

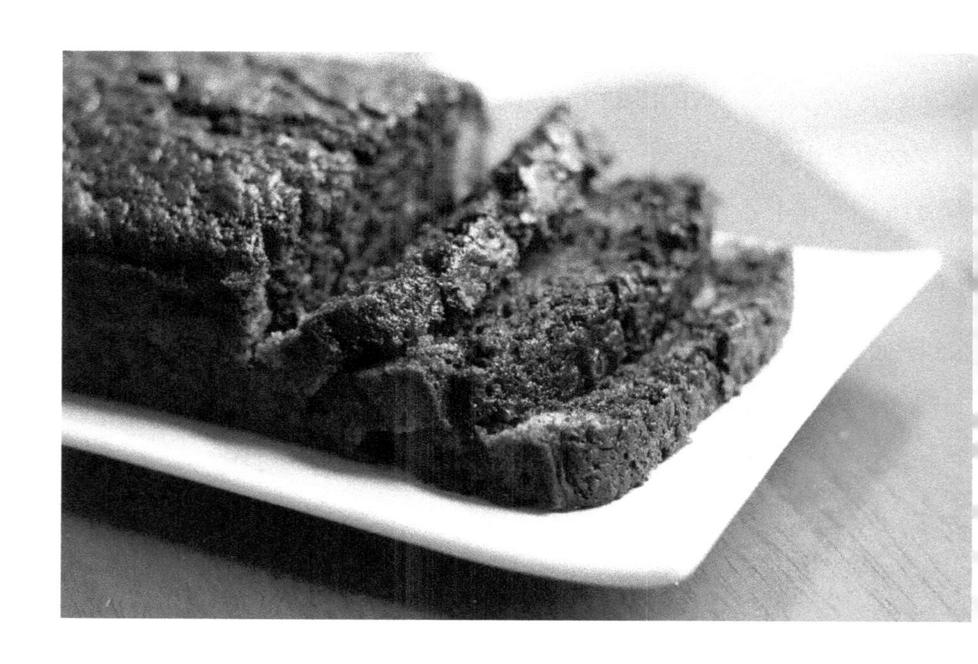

Vegan Pumpkin Bread

Preparation time: 15 minutes Cooking time: 15 minutes
8 Servings.

Ingredients:

1 cup gluten-free flour 1 cup brown rice flour 1 tsp. baking soda ¾ cup brown sugar ½ tsp. baking powder 1 tsp. salt 1 tsp. nutmeg ½ tsp. cinnamon ½ tsp. cloves ½ tsp. allspice 1 cup pumpkin puree ½ cup applesauce 3 tbsp. agave nectar 3 tbsp. water

Directions:

Begin by preheating your oven to 350 degrees Fahrenheit. Next, mix together all the dry ingredients. Next, bring all the wet ingredients together in a different, larger bowl. Pour the dry ingredients into the wet ingredient mixture, and stir well. Pour the batter into a bread pan, and cook the bread for fifty minutes. Allow the bread to cool prior to serving, and enjoy.

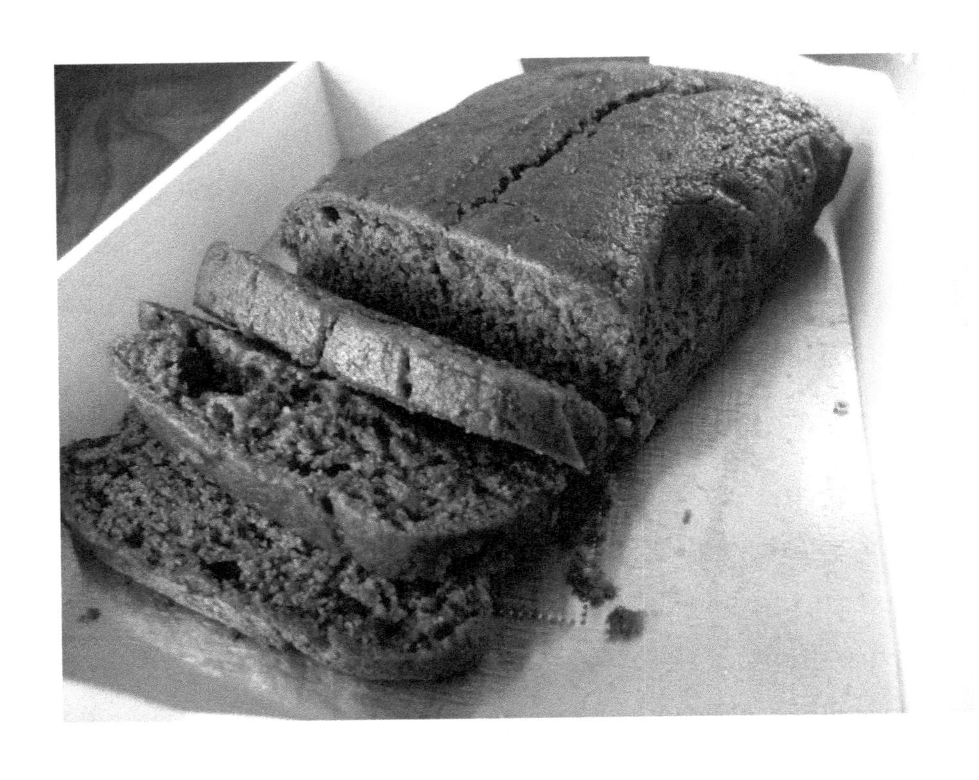

Creative Chocolate "Cream" Pie

Preparation time: 15 minutes Cooking time: 25 minutes 1 pie.

Ingredients:

3 cups all-purpose flour 3 tsp. sugar 1 cup vegan butter 1 tsp. salt 8 tbsp. cold water

Filling ½ cup cornstarch 1/3 cup sugar ½ tsp. salt 3 tbsp. cocoa powder 1 ½ cup almond milk 1 cup coconut milk 1 tsp. vanilla 5 oz. chopped dark chocolate 8 ounces vegan whipped cream

Directions:

Begin by preheating your oven to 425 degrees Fahrenheit. Next, mix together the flour, the sugar, and the salt. Cut the vegan butter into the mixture, making a sort of crumble. Add chilled water in order to make a dough. Roll the dough out in the pie plate. Bake this pie crust for twenty-five minutes. Next, mix together the filling ingredients: from the cornstarch to the vegan whipped cream. Mix well, and then cook the filling in a saucepan over medium heat. Stir continuously. Next, fill the piecrust with the chocolate cream. Cover the pie and chill it in the refrigerator for four hours prior to serving. Enjoy!

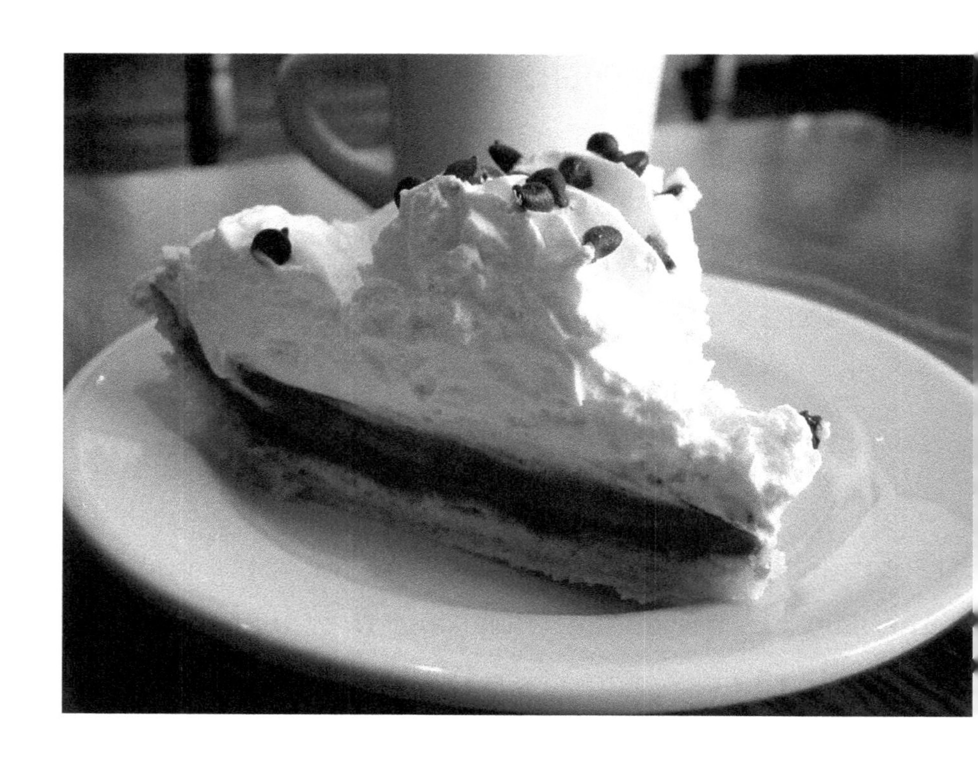

Vegan Apple Cobbler Pie

Preparation time: 15 minutes Cooking time: 25 minutes 6 Pieces.

Ingredients:

3 cups sliced apples 6 cups sliced peaches 2 tbsp. arrowroot powder ½ cup white sugar 1 tsp. cinnamon 1 tsp. vanilla ½ cup water Biscuit Topping Ingredients: ½ cup almond flour 1 cup gluten-free ground-up oats ½ tsp. salt 2 tsp. baking powder 2 tbsp. white sugar 1 tsp. cinnamon ½ cup soymilk 4 tbsp. vegan butter

Directions:

Begin by preheating your oven to 400 degrees Fahrenheit. Next, coat the peaches and the apples with the sugar, arrowroot, the cinnamon, the vanilla, and the water in a large bowl. Allow the mixture to boil in a saucepan. After it begins to boil, allow the apples and peaches to simmer for three minutes. Remove the fruit from the heat and add the vanilla. You've created your base. Now, add the dry ingredients together in a small bowl. Cut the biscuit with the vegan butter to create a crumble. Add the almond milk, and cover the fruit with this batter. Bake this mixture for thirty minutes. Serve warm, and enjoy!

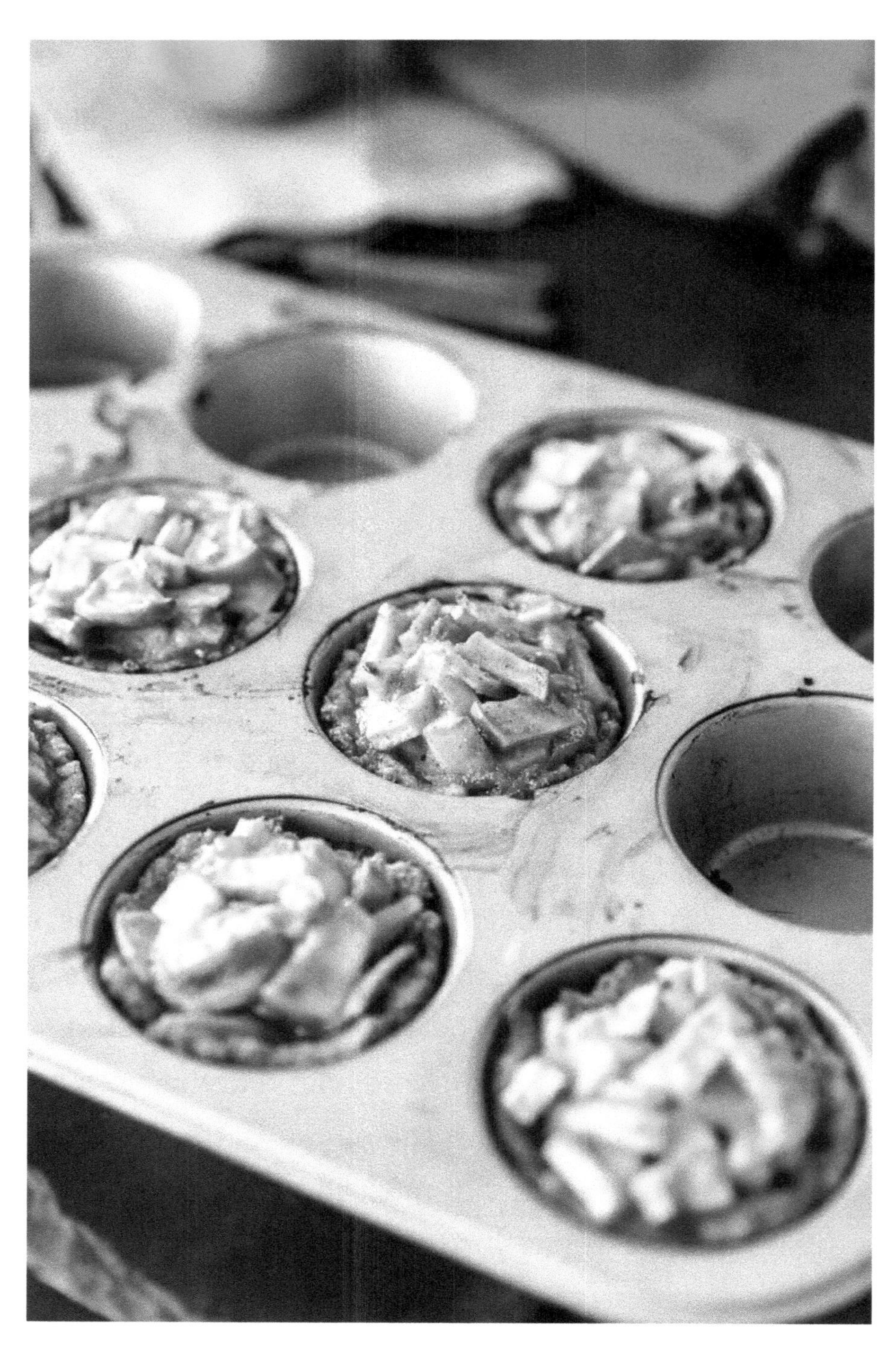

Watermelon Lollies

Preparation time: 15 minutes Cooking time: 35 minutes Servings: 5

Ingredients:

½ cup watermelon, cubed 2 tablespoons lemon juice, freshly squeezed ½ cup water 1 tablespoon stevia

Directions:

In a food processor, put cubed watermelon. Process until smooth. Divide an equal amount of the mixture into an ice pop container. Place inside the freezer for 1 hour. Meanwhile, in a small bowl, put together lemon juice, water, and stevia. Mix well. Pour over frozen watermelon lollies. Add in pop sticks. Freeze for another hour. Pry out watermelon lollies. Serve.

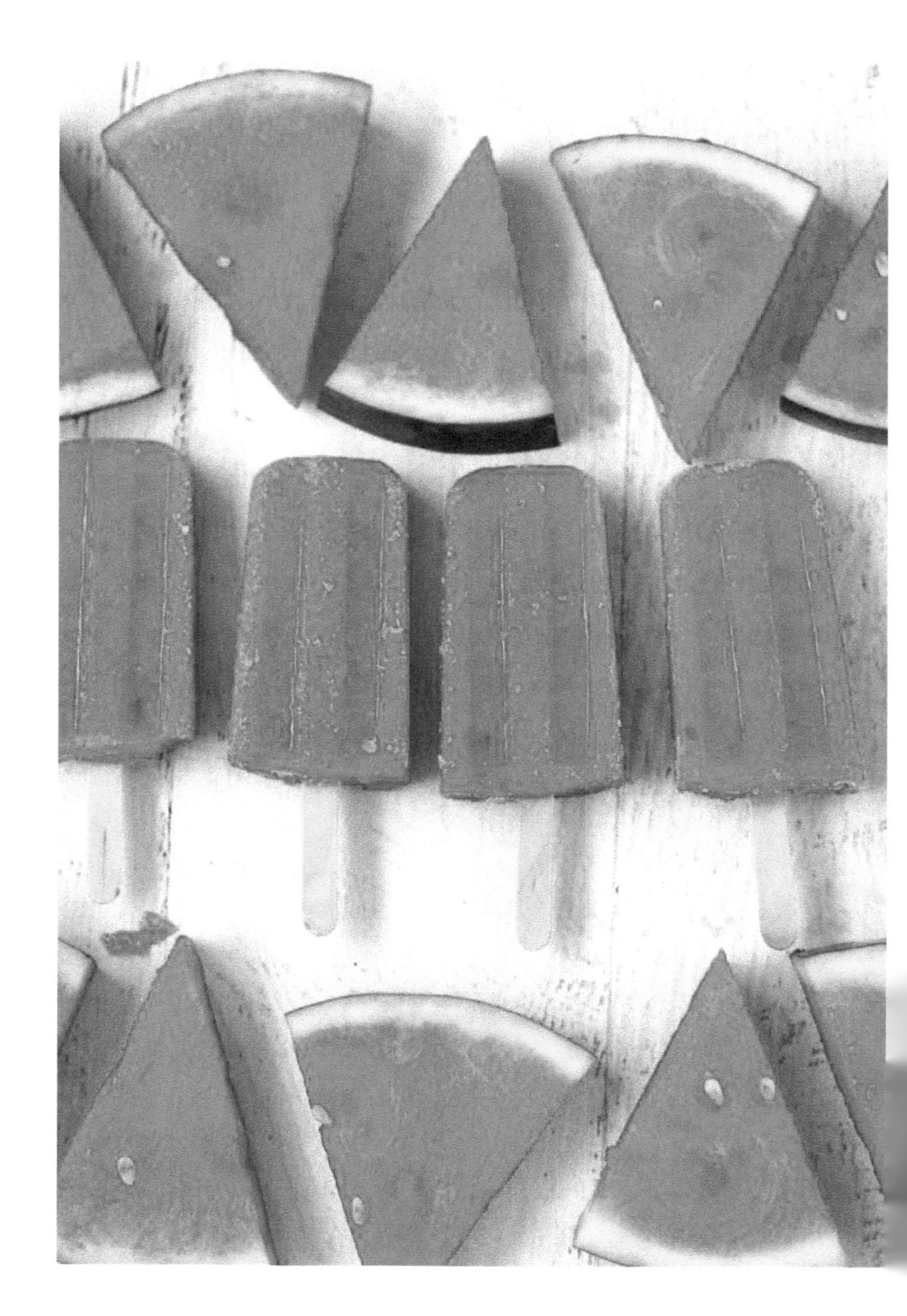

Chocolate Chip Cookies

Preparation time: 15 minutes Cooking time: 45 minutes Servings: 5

Ingredients:

1 ½ cups semisweet vegan chocolate chips 1 tsp baking soda 2 cups flour 1 tsp flax seed 2 tsp vanilla 2/3 cup olive oil ½ tsp salt ¾ cup cocoa powder ½ cup soymilk 1 tbsp flax seed 5 tbsp. Splenda

Directions:

Set the oven at 350 degrees. Place the flax seeds in a blender. Process until it is fine. Add the soy milk and blend for 30 seconds until incorporated. Set it aside. Sift the flour, cocoa, baking soda and salt in a bowl. Cream oil and sugar in a different bowl. Add the soy milk and sugar mixture. Add the vanilla. Mix in the dry ingredients. Add the chocolate chips. Take small dough in your hands and roll it in a ball. Flatten it until it is 1 ½ inch in diameter. Place it in a baking sheet. Make sure to space the balls apart. Bake for 10 minutes. Let it cool for 5 minutes then carefully remove it using a spatula. Transfer it to a cooling rack.

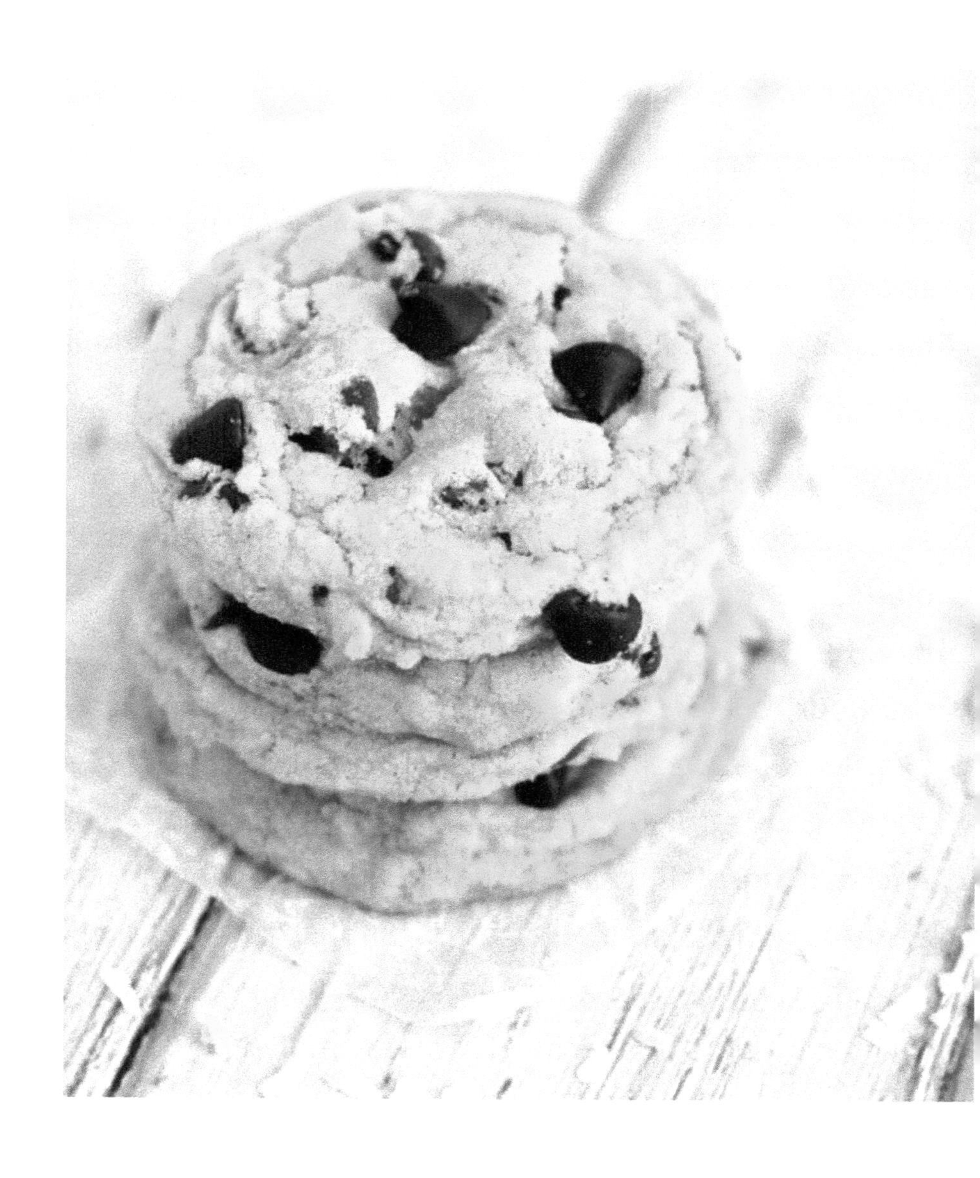

Keto Chocolate Brownies

Preparation time: 15 minutes Cooking time: 35 minutes Servings: 5

Ingredients:

1 1/4 cups almond flour 2/3 cup stevia or coconut sugar 4 1/2 Tbsp cocoa powder 3/4 tsp baking powder 2/3 tsp salt 6 Tbsp melted butter, cooled 5 eggs 1 1/2 tsp pure vanilla extract 2/3 cup 90 percent or pure dark chocolate, chopped

Directions:

Preheat your oven to 350 degrees F. Mix the flour, cocoa powder, stevia or coconut sugar, salt, and baking powder in a mixing bowl. In a separate bowl, beat together the eggs, vanilla, and melted butter. Mix the egg mixture into the flour mixture very well, then stir in the chopped dark chocolate. Pour the mixture into a baking pan and bake for 30 to 40 minutes. To check, poke the center with a toothpick, and if it comes out clean then it is ready. Set on a cooling rack for 7 minutes, then slice into 12 pieces and serve.

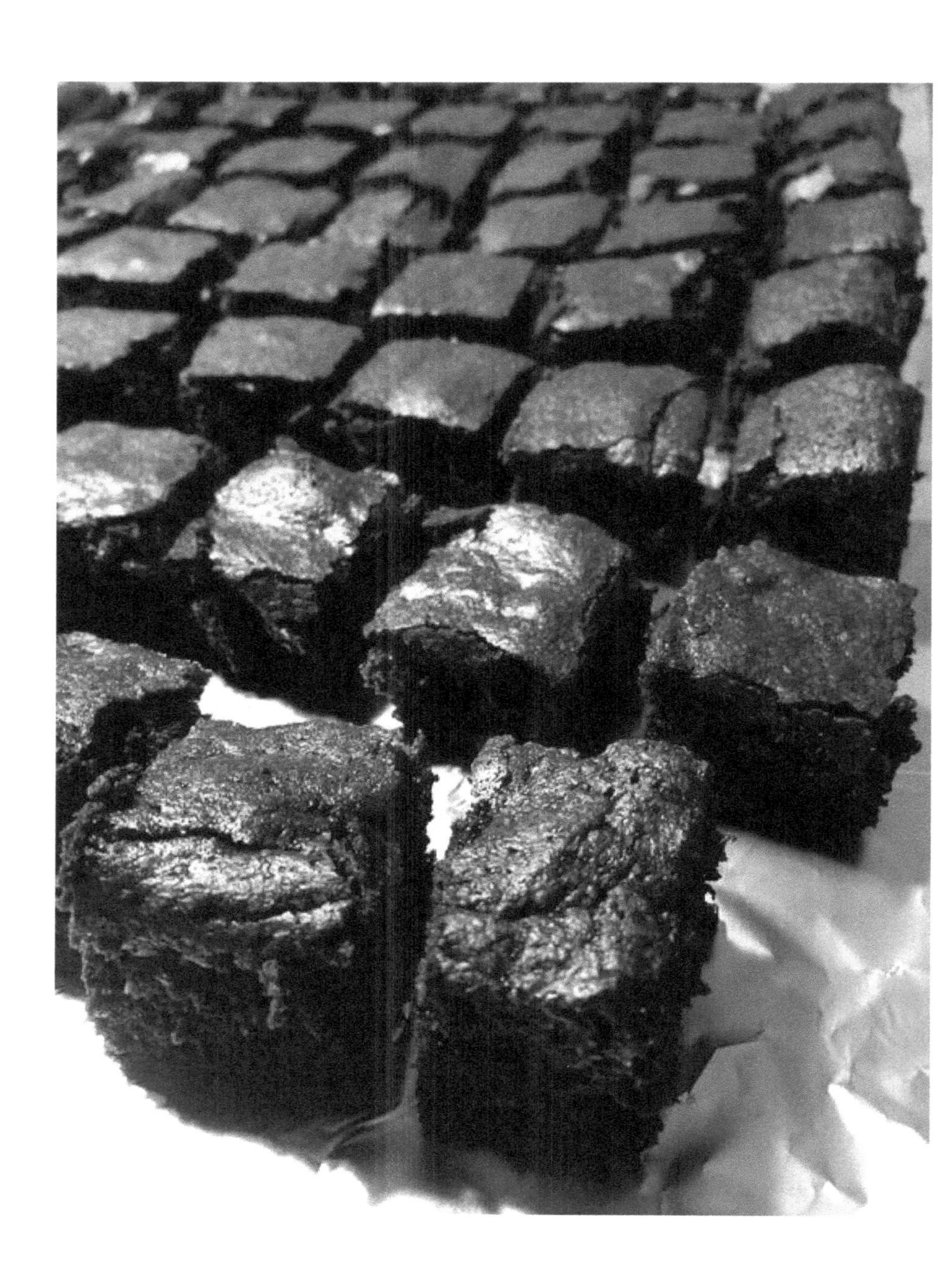

Orange Blueberry Blast

Preparation time: 30 minutes Cooking time: 0 minutes Servings: 01

Ingredients:

1 cup almond milk 1 scoop plant-based protein powder 1 cup blueberries 1 orange, peeled 1 teaspoon nutmeg 1 tablespoon shredded coconut

Directions:

Add all ingredients to a blender. Hit the pulse button and blend till it is smooth. Chill well to serve.

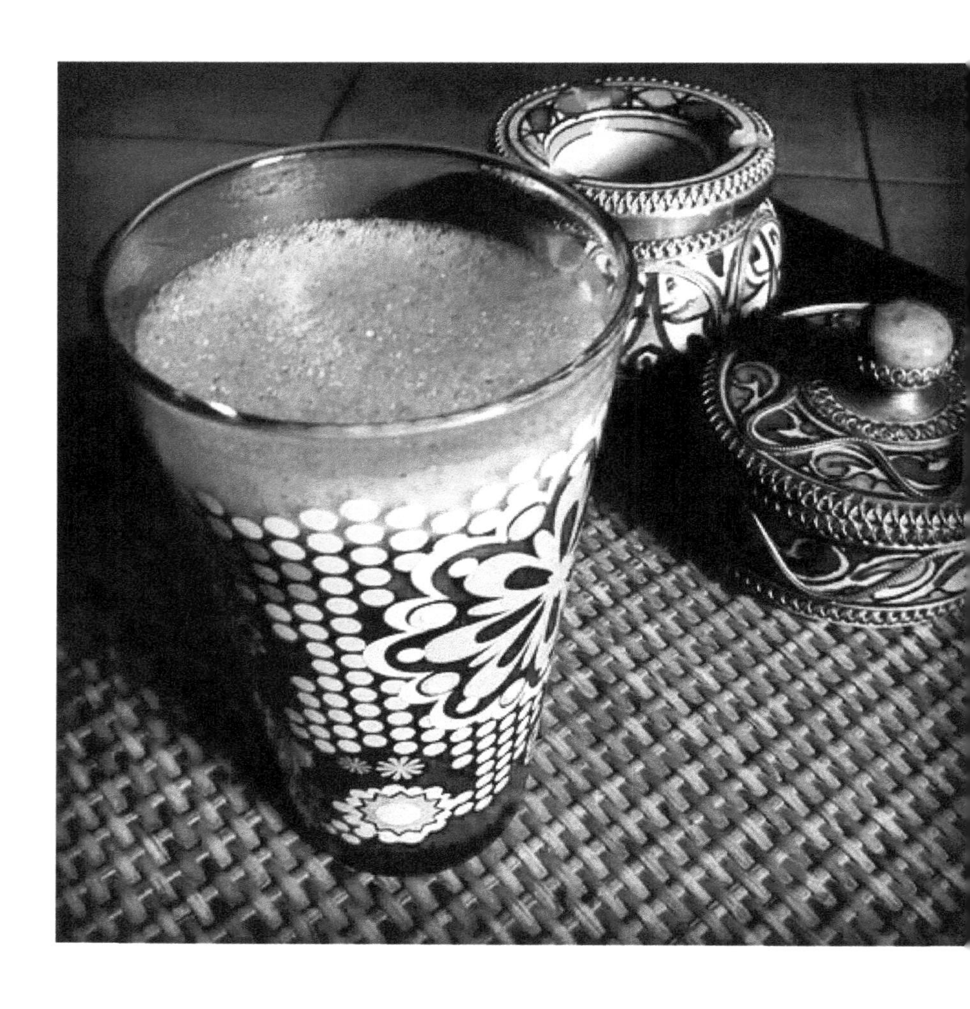

Chocolate coconut almond tart

Preparation time: 15 minutes | Cooking time: 25 minutes | Servings: 8-10

Ingredients:

For crust:

1 cup almonds 2 tbsp. maple syrup 1 cup almond flour 3 tbsp. coconut oil

Filling & topping:

3 oz. bittersweet chocolate bars 1 tbsp. maple syrup 13.5 oz. coconut milk Coconut, almonds Sea salt a pinch

Directions: In a blender mix the almond flour and almonds until chopped and mix evenly. Pour maple syrup and coconut oil or mix well. Pour the batter into a baking pan and press it with a spoon to set its edges. Bake the pie for 10 to 1 minutes in a preheated oven at 300 degrees until golden brown. Take a medium bowl, add chocolate and melt it over the boiling water. Add maple syrup on the top of the chocolate. In a pan, add coconut milk and boil on a flame, pour the chocolate in boiling coconut milk and stir well until smooth. Now pour the filling on the crust and top with almonds, coconut and sea salt. Store in a refrigerator for 2 hours or leave over the night. Serve the tart when completely set.

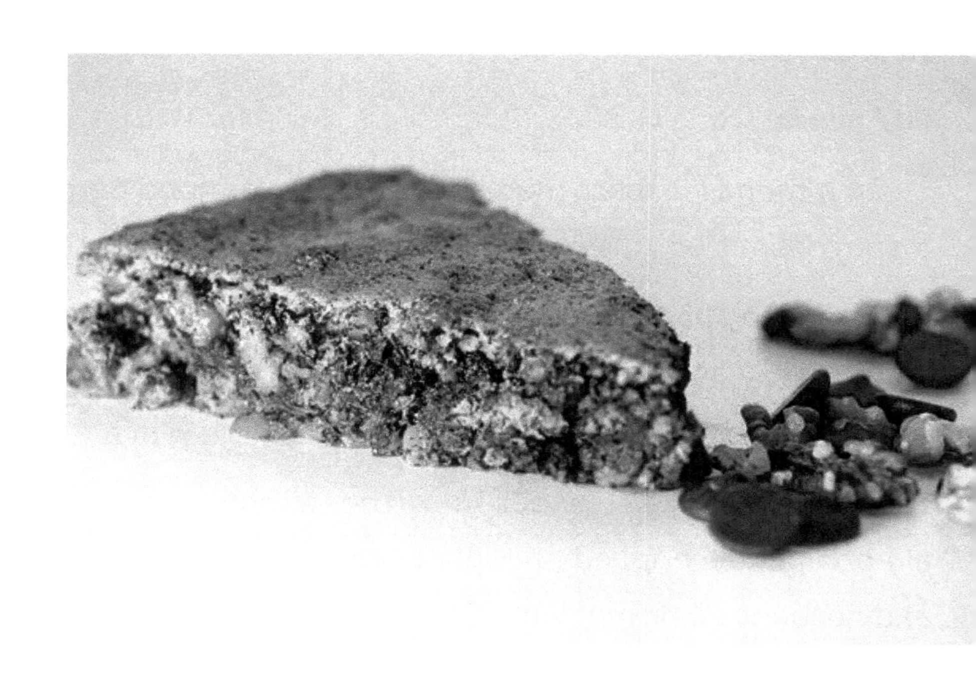

Peanut butter and celery

Preparation time: 5 minutes | Cooking time: 5 minutes | Servings: 2

Ingredients:

4 stalks celery 1 cup peanut butter

Directions: Take 4 stalks of celery, clean them well and let it dry. Now cut one stalk in 3 equal parts. Apply the peanut butter with the knife on every stalk piece. Serve it with a cold glass of milk or enjoy a crunchy peanut butter celery.

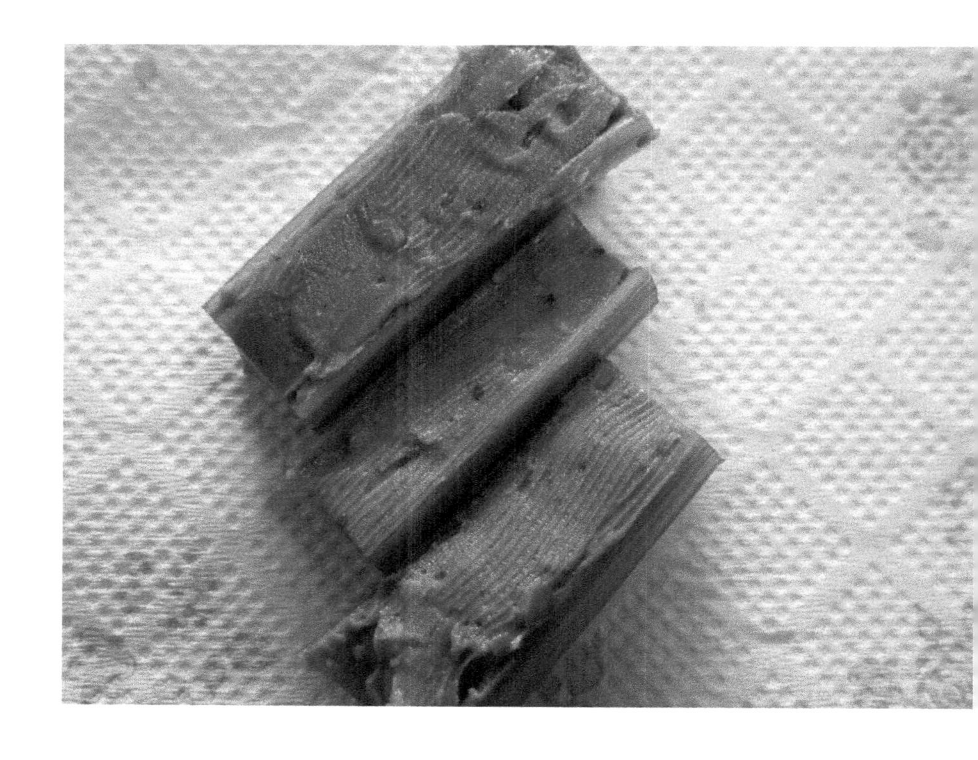

Chewy lemon oatmeal cookies

Preparation time: 25 minutes | Cooking time: 45 minutes | Servings: 14-16 cookies

Ingredients:

10 dates 1 cup oats 1 cup applesauce 1 cup oat flour 1 ½ tsp apple cider vinegar ½ cup cooking oats ¾ cup chopped walnuts 2 tbsp. lemon zest 2 tsp cocoa powder 1 tsp vanilla powder ½ tsp baking soda Sea salt a pinch

Directions:

Take a small bowl, fill it with water and soak dates for 20 minutes. Preheat oven at 275 degrees. Strain the excessive water from dates and pour them into the blender, add applesauce and vinegar and blend well until turn into a paste. Take a large bowl, mix oats, oat flour, cooking oats, walnuts, lemon zest, cocoa powder, vanilla powder, baking soda, and salt. Now add the dates paste into the mixture and stir well. Take a small amount of the mixture on hands, make small balls and flatten them with hand. Place them onto the baking sheet. Bake the cookies for almost 35 to 45 minutes until they turn brown and crispy. Let them cool and serve. You can store them for 4 to 5 days at room temperature.

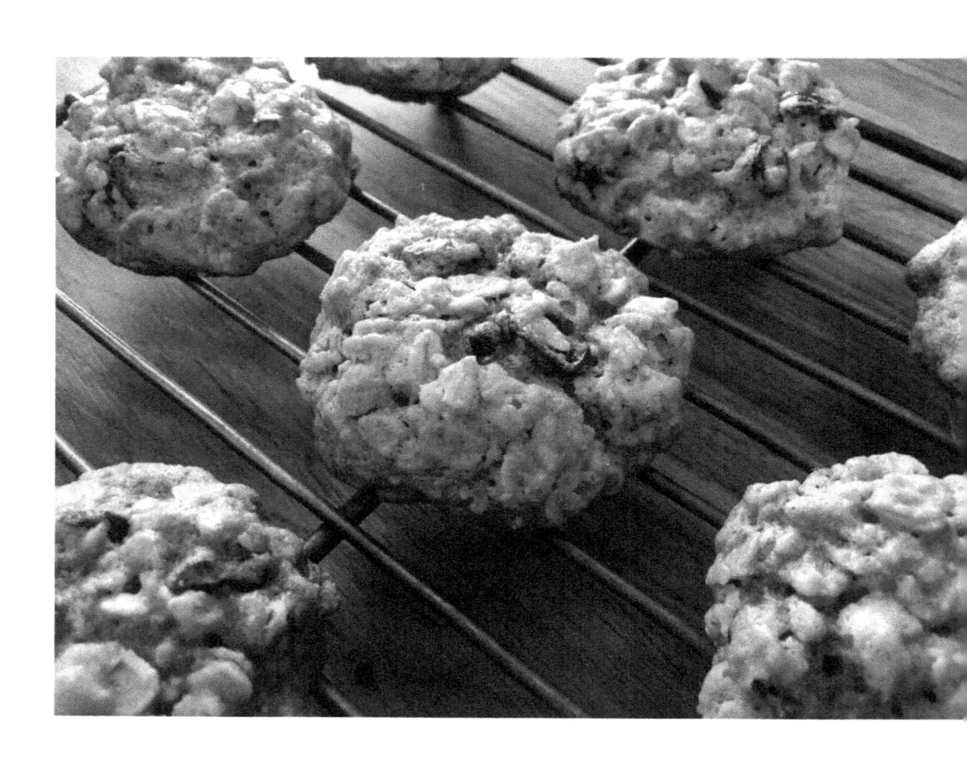

Pumpkin Fig Smoothie

Preparation time: 30 minutes Cooking time: 0 minutes Servings: 01

Ingredients:

½ large frozen banana 3 fresh figs ⅓ cup canned pumpkin 2 tablespoons almond butter 1 cup almond milk 3 ice cubes 1 tablespoon hemp hearts

Directions:

Add all ingredients to a blender. Hit the pulse button and blend till it is smooth. Chill well to serve.

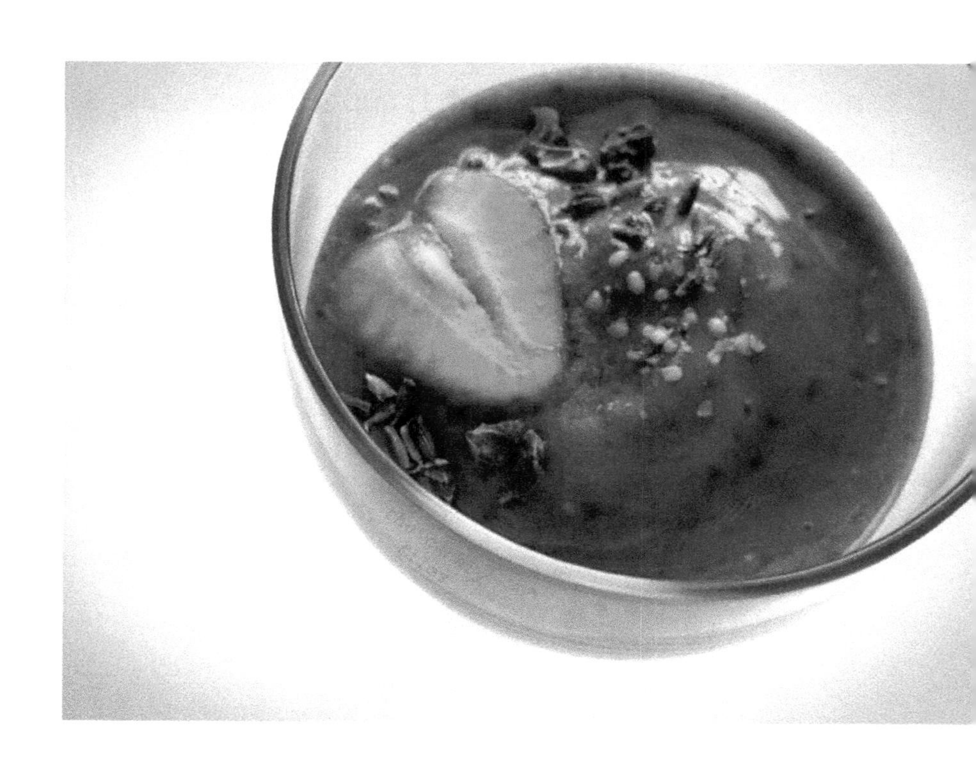

Homemade Apricot and Soy Nut Trail Mix

Preparation time: 15 minutes Cooking time: 0 minutes Servings: 20

Ingredients:

¼ cup dried apricots, chopped 1 cup pumpkin seeds ½ cup roasted cashew nuts 1 cup roasted, shelled pistachios What you'll need from the store cupboard: Salt to taste 3 tbsp MCT oil or coconut oil

Directions

In a medium mixing bowl, place all ingredients. Thoroughly combine. Bake in the oven for 10 minutes at 3750F. In 20 small zip-top bags, get ¼ cup of the mixture and place in each bag. One zip-top bag is equal to one serving. If properly stored, this can last up to two weeks.

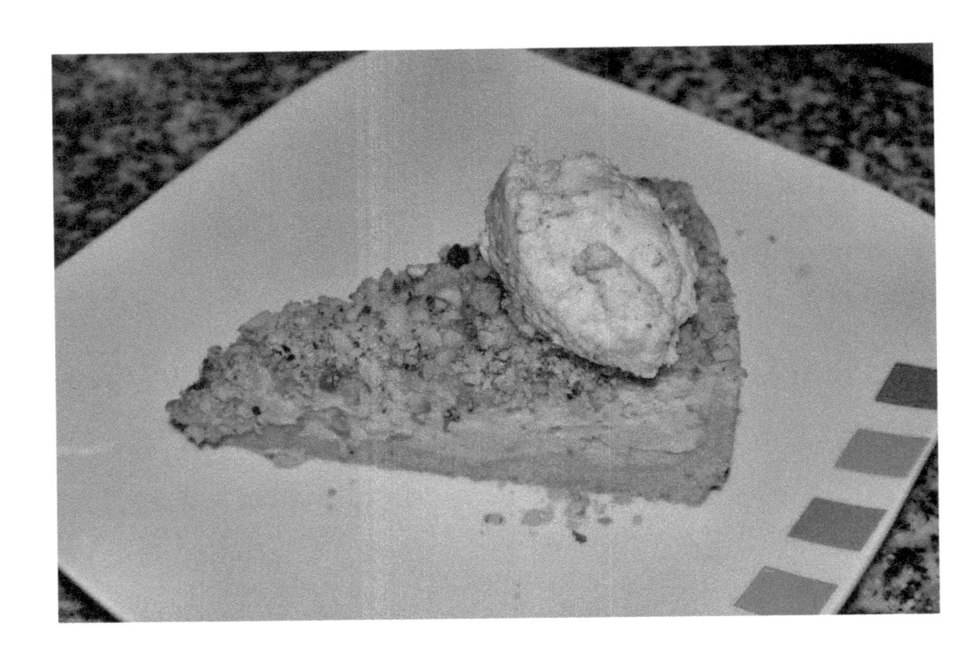

Oatmeal Cinnamon Bars

Preparation time: 15 minutes Cooking time: 35 minutes 12 bars.

Ingredients:

1 tbsp. ground flax 3 tbsp. water 1 tsp. vanilla 1 cup coconut sugar 1/3 cup coconut oil ½ tsp. baking soda 1 tsp. vanilla 1 tsp. cinnamon 1 cup ground rolled oats (in food processor) 1 cup oats 1 cup almond flour 1/3 cup nondairy chocolate chips

Directions: Begin by preheating the oven to 350 degrees Fahrenheit. Next, mix together the flax seeds and the water and set them to the side for five minutes. Beat together the sugar and the coconut oil with beaters. Next, add the flax egg and the vanilla and continue to beat. Add the soda, salt, and the cinnamon, and continue to beat. Lastly, add the dry ingredients and beat the mixture until it's perfectly combined. Next, spread the dough into a baking pan and layer the chocolate chips overtop. Press them into the pan. Bake the cookie for twenty minutes. Afterwards, allow the cookies to cool. Slice them up and serve them. Enjoy!

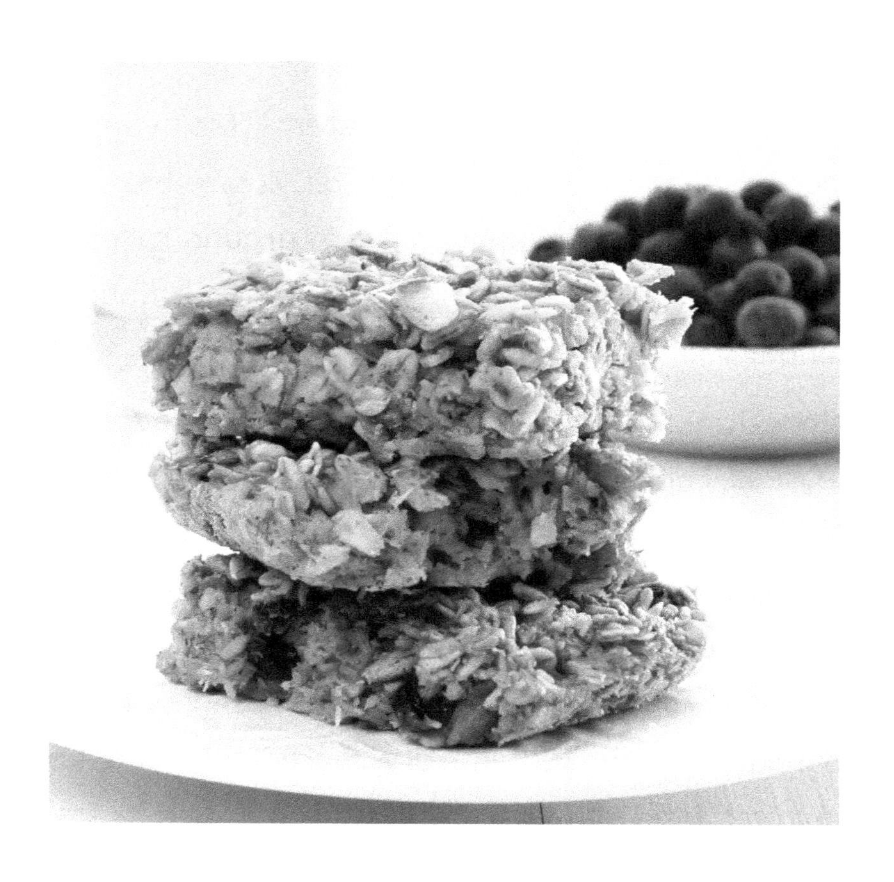

Infused water

Preparation time: 5 minutes Cooking time: 20 minutes Servings: 12

Ingredients:

1 lemon 1 orange 1 tbsp fresh ginger 5 cardamom pods ¼ tsp peppercorn 1 cinnamon stick 6 cups water

Directions:

Cut orange and lemon into slices and smash the cardamom pods. Peel the ginger and slice it up. Add all ingredients to a pot and bring to a boil. Once boiling, stir and reduce the heat to a simmer. Let it simmer until the fruit slices break down. Strain the liquid into a glass and serve with sugar if desired.

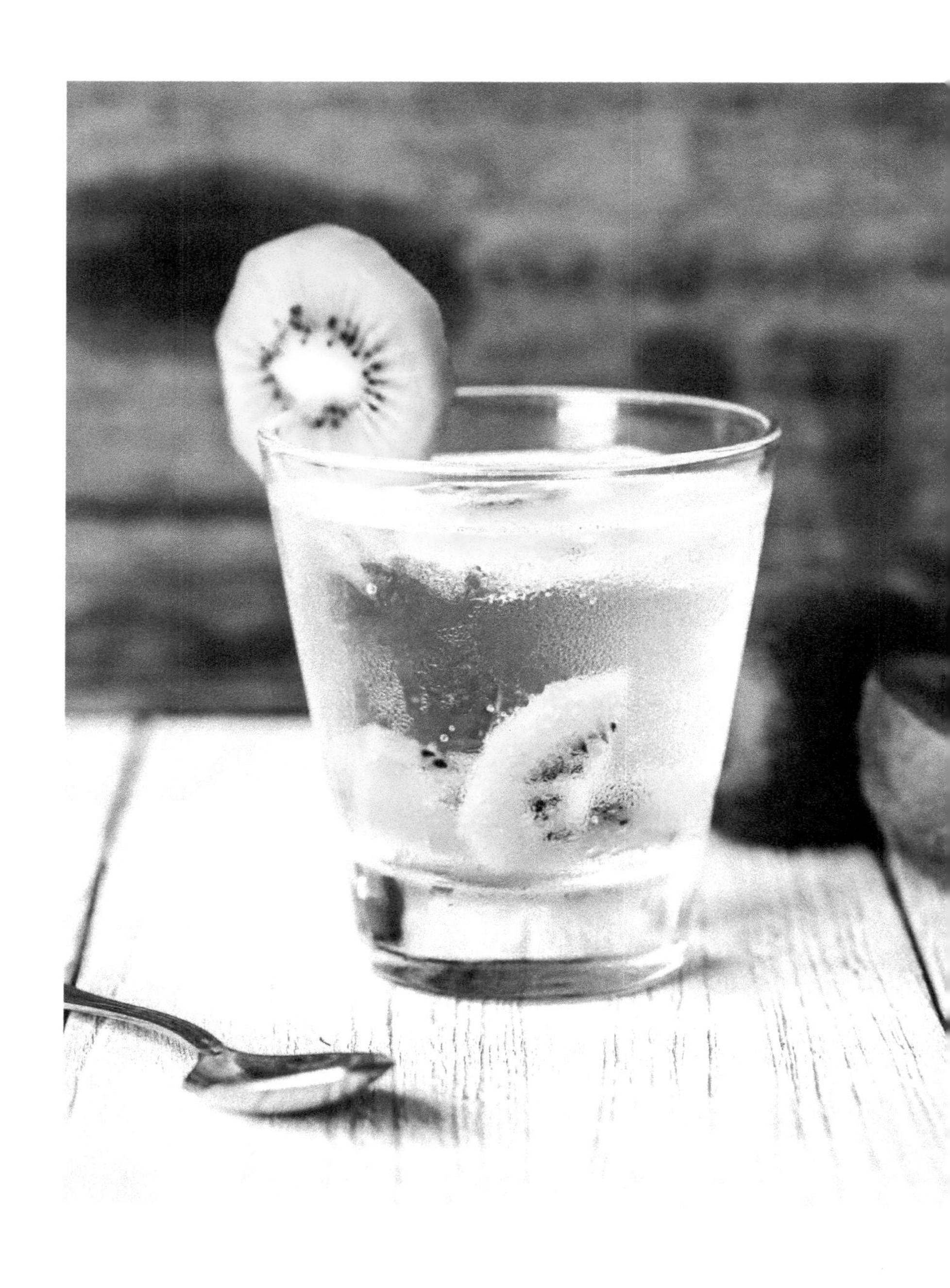

Almond Choco Shake

Preparation time: 5 minutes Cooking time: 0 minutes Servings: 1

Ingredients:

½ cup heavy cream, liquid 1 tbsp cocoa powder 1 packet Stevia, or more to taste 5 almonds, chopped What you'll need from the store cupboard: 1 ½ cups water 3 tbsp coconut oil

Directions

Add all ingredients in a blender. Blend until smooth and creamy. Serve and enjoy.

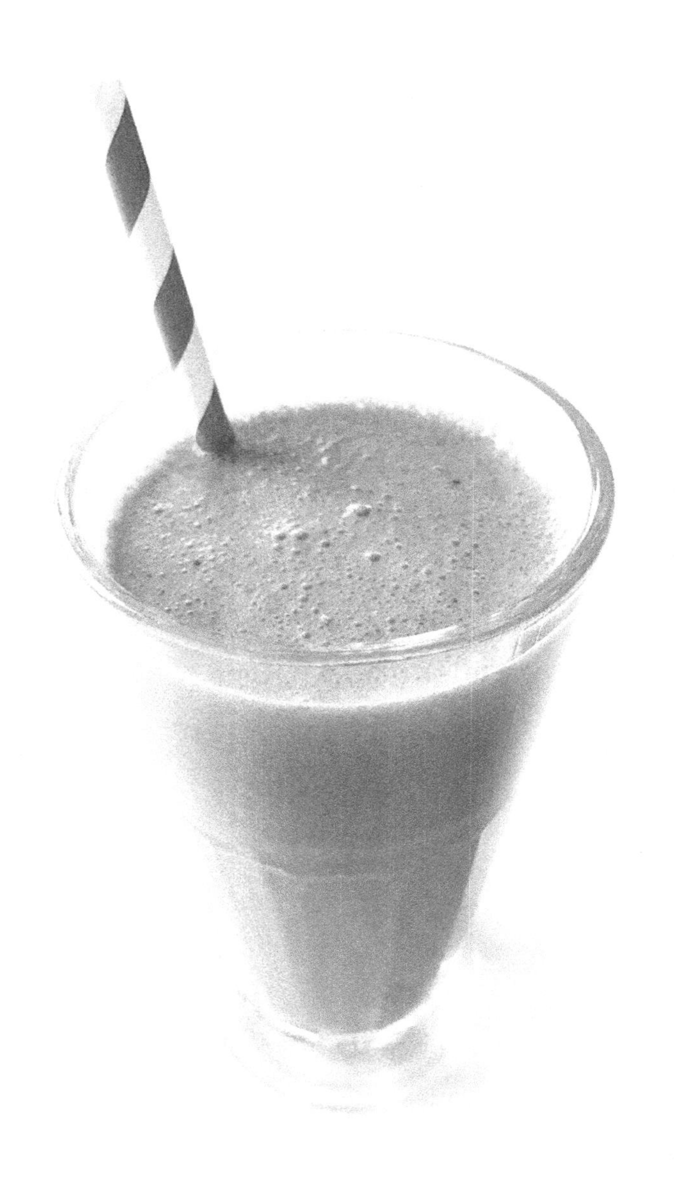

Raspberry-Choco Shake

Preparation time: 5 minutes Cooking time: 0 minutes Servings: 1

Ingredients:

¼ cup heavy cream, liquid 1 tbsp cocoa powder 1 packet Stevia, or more to taste ¼ cup raspberries What you'll need from the store cupboard: 1 ½ cups water

Directions

Add all ingredients in a blender. Blend until smooth and creamy. Serve and enjoy.

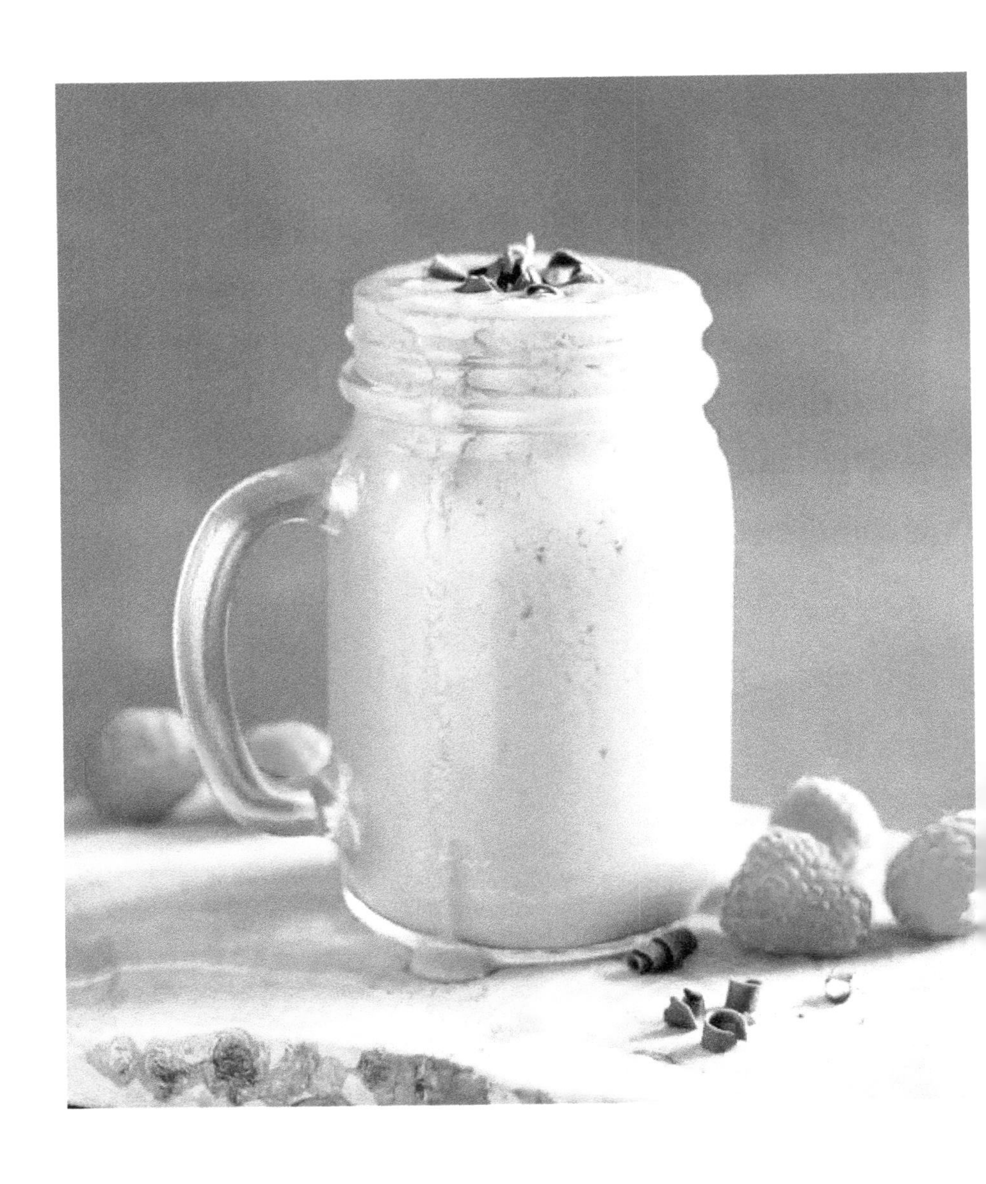

Spiced Almond Shake

Preparation time: 5 minutesCooking time: 0 minutes Servings: 1

Ingredients:

½ cup coconut milk 1 tbsp cocoa powder ¼ cup almonds, sliced ¼ tsp allspice 1 tbsp almond oil What you'll need from the store cupboard: 1 packet Stevia, or more to taste 1 cup water ½ tsp cinnamon ¼ tsp nutmeg 3 tablespoons olive oil

Directions Add all ingredients in a mixer. Whisk until smooth and creamy. Serve and enjoy.

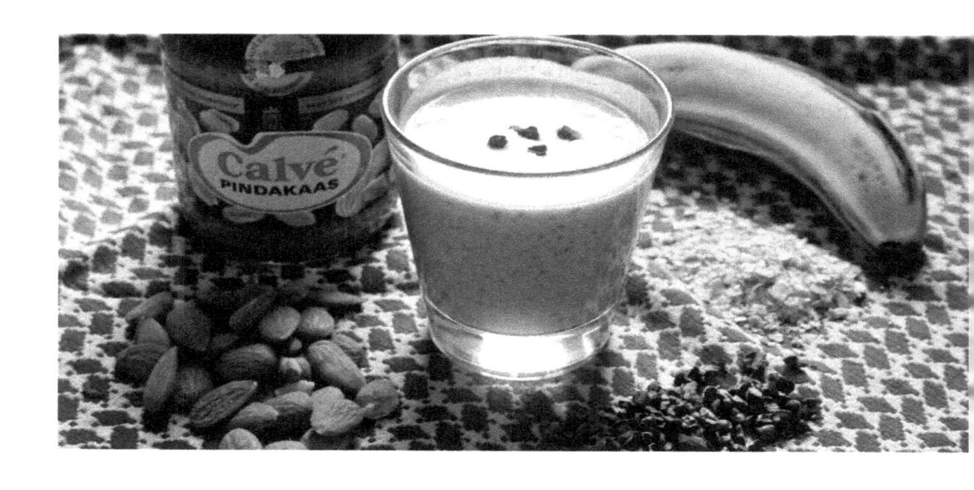
Calvé
PINDAKAAS

Rich Truffle Hot Chocolate

Servings: 4 Preparation time: 1 hours and 10 minutes

Ingredients:

1/3 cup of cocoa powder, unsweetened 1/3 cup of coconut sugar 1/8 teaspoon of salt 1/8 teaspoon of ground cinnamon 1 teaspoon of vanilla extract, unsweetened 32 fluid ounce of coconut milk

Directions: Using a 2 quarts slow cooker, add all the ingredients and stir properly. Cover it with the lid, then plug in the slow cooker and cook it for 2 hours on the high heat setting or until it is heated thoroughly. When done, serve right away.

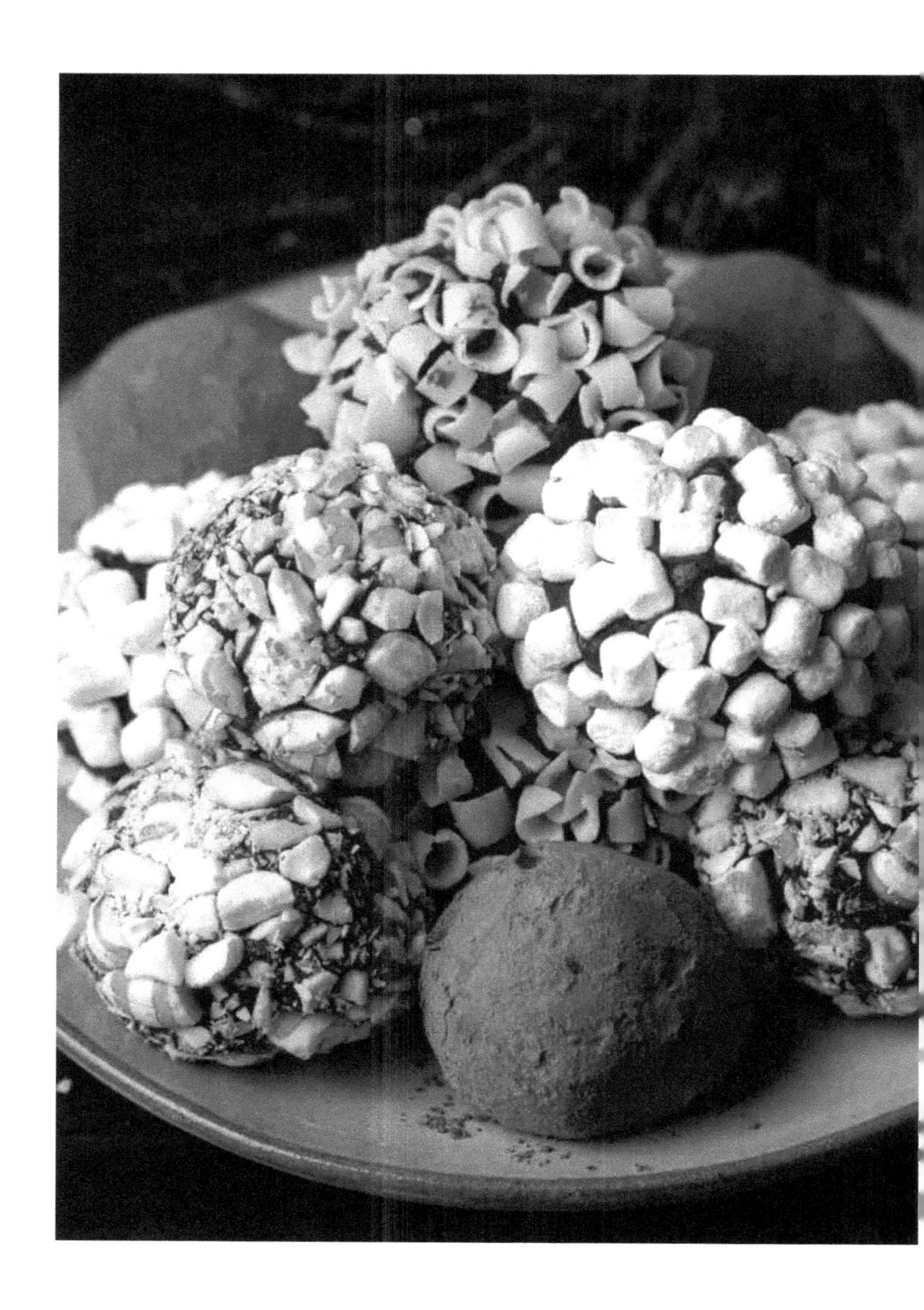

Nutty Choco Milk Shake

Preparation time: 5 minutes Cooking time: 0 minutes Servings: 1

Ingredients:

¼ cup half and half 1 tbsp cocoa powder 1 packet Stevia, or more to taste 4 pecans 1 tbsp macadamia oil What you'll need from the store cupboard: 1 ½ cups water 3 tbsp coconut oil

Directions

Add all ingredients in a blender. Blend until smooth and creamy. Serve and enjoy.

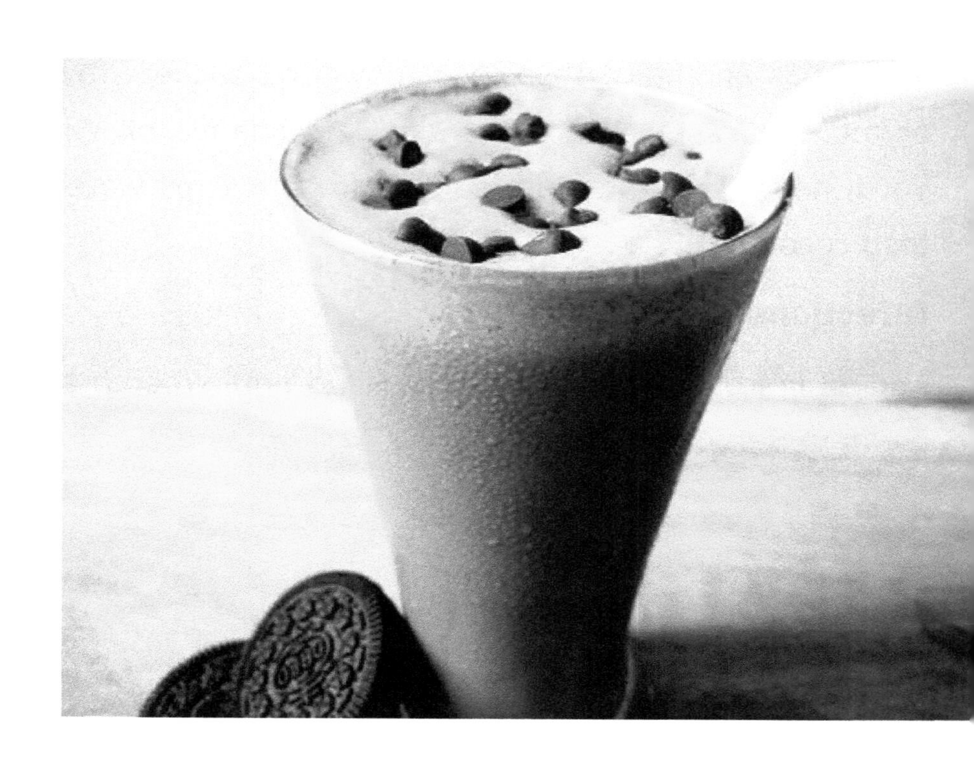

Avocado and Greens Smoothie

Preparation time: 5 minutes Cooking time: 0 minutes Servings: 1

Ingredients:

½ cup coconut milk ¼ avocado fruit ½ cup spring mix greens 3 tbsps avocado oil What you'll need from the store cupboard: 1 ½ cups water 2 packets Stevia, or as needed

Directions

Add all ingredients in a blender. Blend until smooth and creamy. Serve and enjoy.

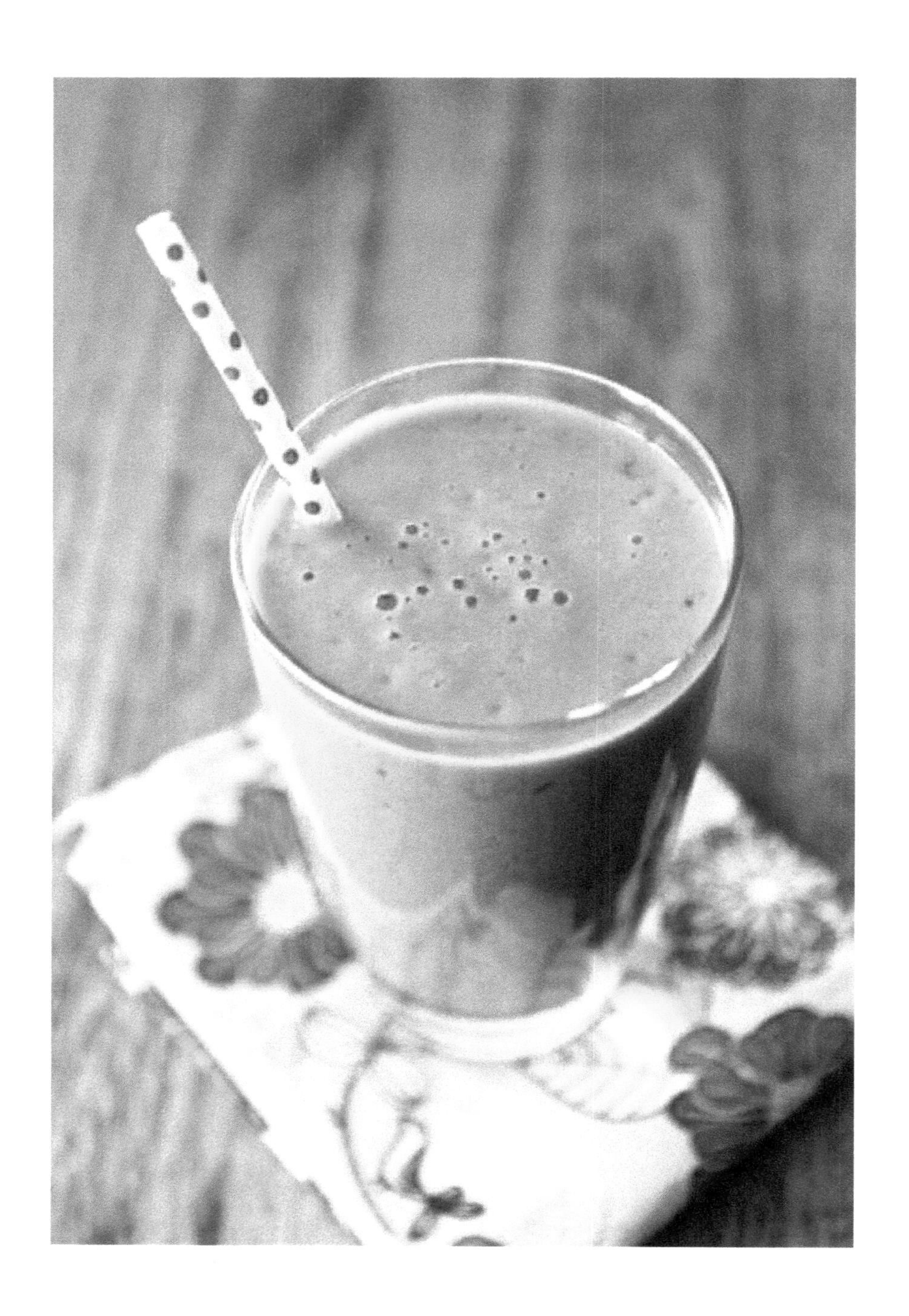

Chocolate and Avocado Pudding

Preparation time:3 hours and 10 minutes Cooking time:0 minute Servings: 1

Ingredients:

1 small avocado, pitted, peeled 1 small banana, mashed 1/3 cup cocoa powder, unsweetened 1 tablespoon cacao nibs, unsweetened 1/4 cup maple syrup 1/3 cup coconut cream

Directions:

Add avocado in a food processor along with cream and then pulse for 2 minutes until smooth. Add remaining ingredients, blend until mixed, and then tip the pudding in a container. Cover the container with a plastic wrap; it should touch the pudding and refrigerate for 3 hours. Serve straight away.

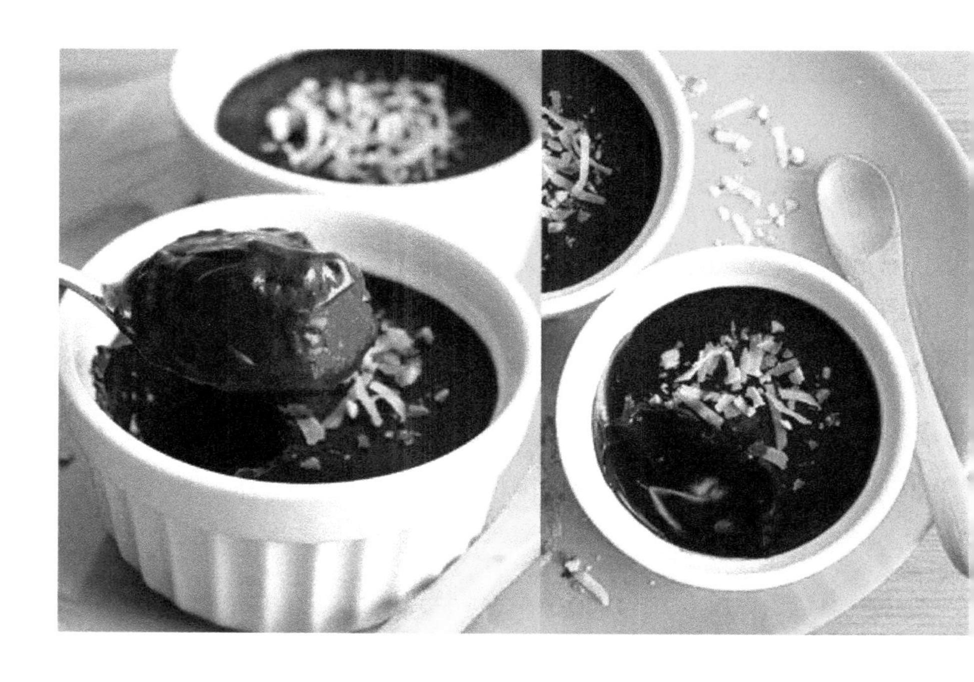

Watermelon Mint Popsicles

Preparation time: 8 hours and 5 minutes Cooking time: 0 minute Servings: 8

Ingredients:

20 mint leaves, diced 6 cups watermelon chunks 3 tablespoons lime juice

Directions:

Add watermelon in a food processor along with lime juice and then pulse for 15 seconds until smooth. Pass the watermelon mixture through a strainer placed over a bowl, remove the seeds and then stir mint into the collected watermelon mixture. Take eight Popsicle molds, pour in prepared watermelon mixture, and freeze for 2 hours until slightly firm. Then insert popsicle sticks and continue freezing for 6 hours until solid. Serve straight away

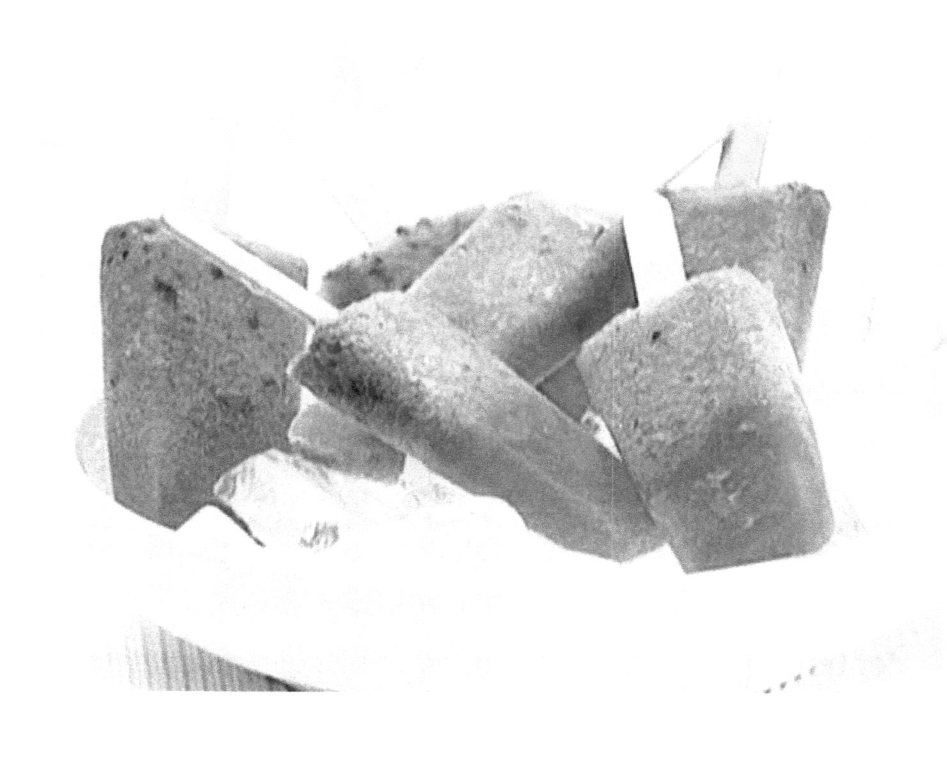

Brownie Energy Bites

Preparation time: 1 hour and 10 minutes Cooking time: 0 minute Servings: 2

Ingredients:

1/2 cup walnuts 1 cup Medjool dates, chopped 1/2 cup almonds 1/8 teaspoon salt 1/2 cup shredded coconut flakes 1/3 cup and 2 teaspoons cocoa powder, unsweetened

Directions:

Place almonds and walnuts in a food processor and pulse for 3 minutes until the dough starts to come together. Add remaining ingredients, reserving ¼ cup of coconut and pulse for 2 minutes until incorporated. Shape the mixture into balls, roll them in remaining coconut until coated, and refrigerate for 1 hour. Serve straight away

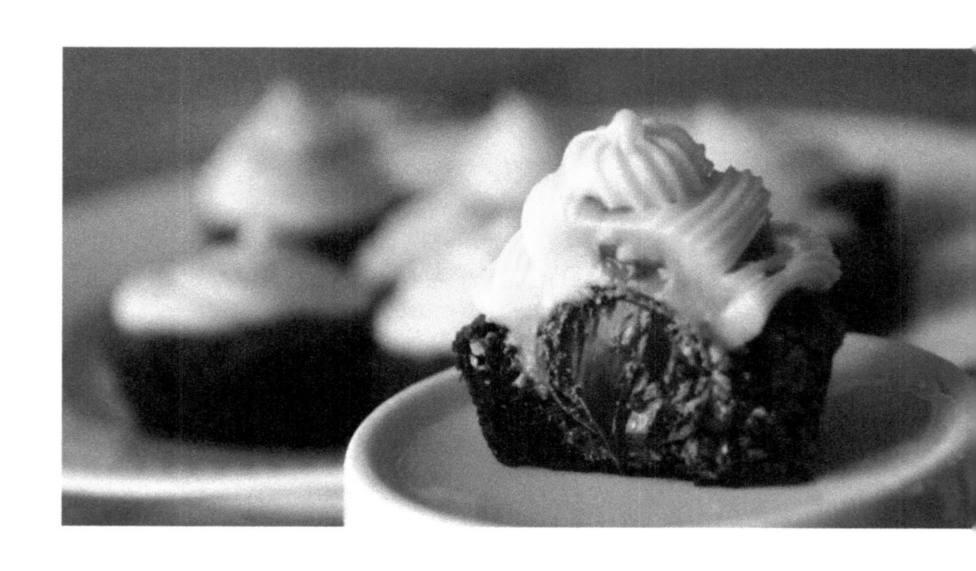

Salted Caramel Chocolate Cups

Preparation time: 5 minutes Cooking time: 2 minutes Servings: 12

Ingredients:

¼ teaspoon sea salt granules 1 cup dark chocolate chips, unsweetened 2 teaspoons coconut oil 6 tablespoons caramel sauce

Directions:

Take a heatproof bowl, add chocolate chips and oil, stir until mixed, then microwave for 1 minute until melted, stir chocolate and continue heating in the microwave for 30 seconds. Take twelve mini muffin tins, line them with muffin liners, spoon a little bit of chocolate mixture into the tins, spread the chocolate in the bottom and along the sides, and freeze for 10 minutes until set. Then fill each cup with ½ tablespoon of caramel sauce, cover with remaining chocolate and freeze for another 2salt0 minutes until set. When ready to eat, peel off liner from the cup, sprinkle with sauce, and serve.

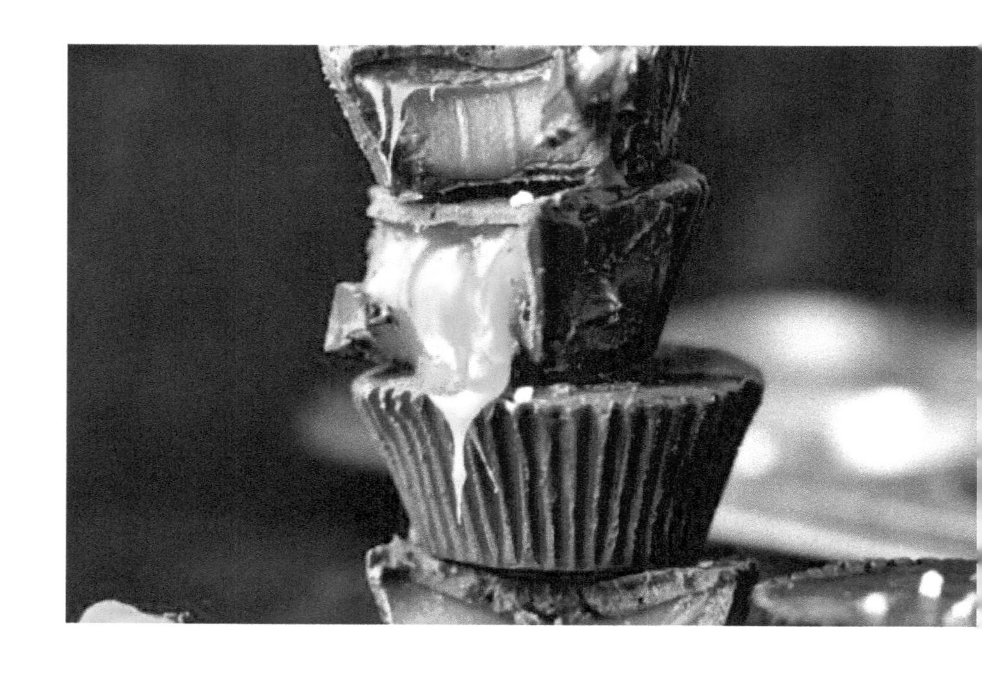

Mango Coconut Cheesecake

Preparation time:4 hours and 10 minutes Cooking time:0 minute Servings: 4

Ingredients:

For the Crust: 1 cup macadamia nuts 1 cup dates, pitted, soaked in hot water for 10 minutes

For the Filling: 2 cups cashews, soaked in warm water for 10 minutes 1/2 cup and 1 tablespoon maple syrup 1/3 cup and 2 tablespoons coconut oil 1/4 cup lemon juice 1/2 cup and 2 tablespoons coconut milk, unsweetened, chilled

For the Topping: 1 cup fresh mango slices

Directions:

Prepare the crust, and for this, place nuts in a food processor and process until mixture resembles crumbs. Drain the dates, add them to the food processor and blend for 2 minutes until thick mixture comes together. Take a 4-inch cheesecake pan, place date mixture in it, spread and press evenly, and set aside. Prepare the filling and for this, place all its ingredients in a food processor and blend for 3 minutes until smooth. Pour the filling into the crust, spread evenly, and then freeze for 4 hours until set. Top the cake with mango slices and then serve.

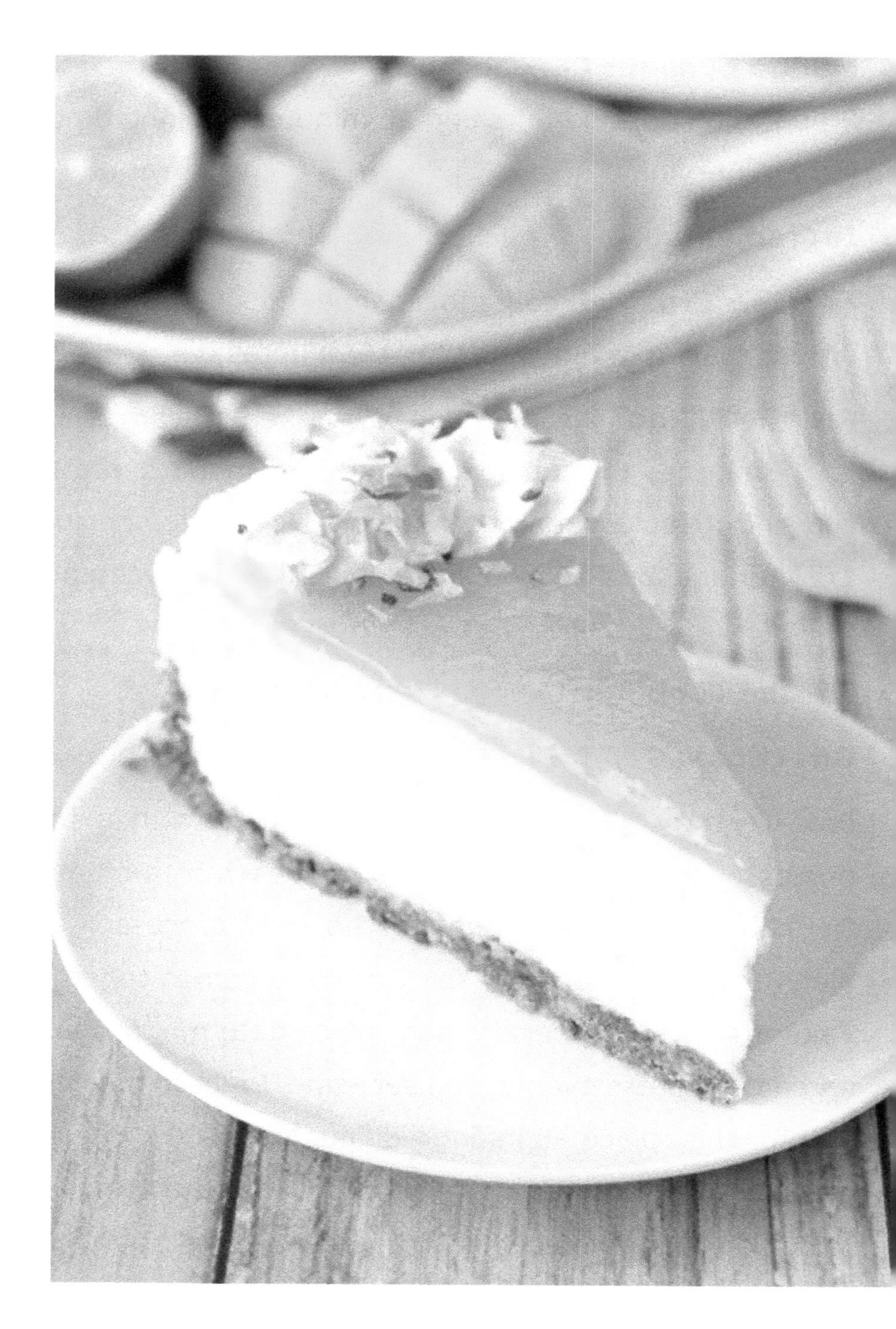

Cookie Dough Bites

Preparation time:4 hours and10 minutes Cooking time:0 minuteServings: 18

Ingredients:

15 ounces cooked chickpeas 1/3 cup vegan chocolate chips 1/3 cup and 2 tablespoons peanut butter 8 Medjool dates pitted 1 teaspoon vanilla extract, unsweetened 2 tablespoons maple syrup 1 1/2 tablespoons almond milk, unsweetened

Directions:

Place chickpeas in a food processor along with dates, butter, and vanilla and then process for 2 minutes until smooth. Add remaining ingredients, except for chocolate chips, and then pulse for 1 minute until blends and dough comes together. Add chocolate chips, stir until just mixed, then shape the mixture into 18 balls and refrigerate for 4 hours until firm. Serve straight away

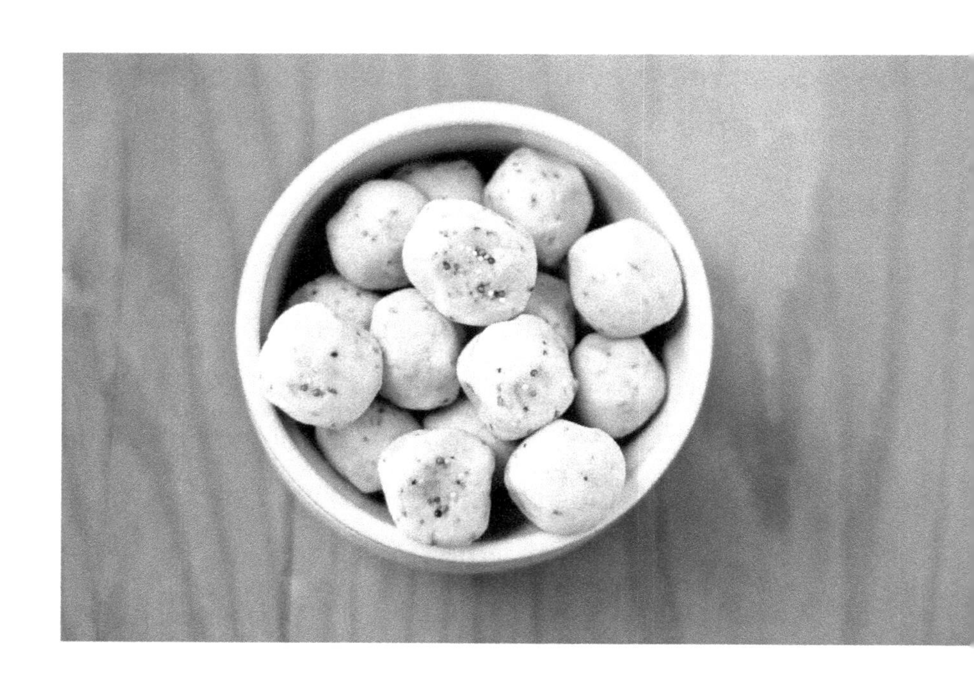

Almond Butter, Oat and Protein Energy Balls

Preparation time:1 hour and 10 minutes Cooking time: 3 minutesServings: 4

Ingredients:

1 cup rolled oats ½ cup honey 2 ½ scoops of vanilla protein powder 1 cup almond butter Chia seeds for rolling

Directions:

Take a skillet pan, place it over medium heat, add butter and honey, stir and cook for 2 minutes until warm. Transfer the mixture into a bowl, stir in protein powder until mixed, and then stir in oatmeal until combined. Shape the mixture into balls, roll them into chia seeds, then arrange them on a cookie sheet and refrigerate for 1 hour until firm. Serve straight away

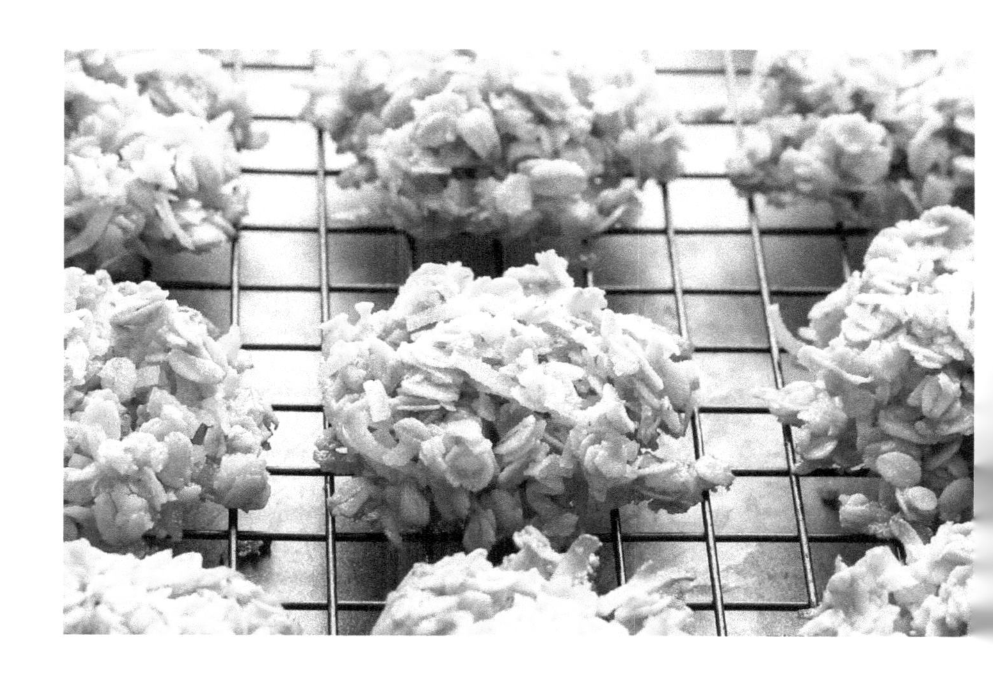

Coconut Oil Cookies

Preparation time: 10 minutes Cooking time: 10 minutes Servings: 15

Ingredients:

3 1/4 cup oats 1/2 teaspoons salt 2 cups coconut Sugar 1 teaspoons vanilla extract, unsweetened 1/4 cup cocoa powder 1/2 cup liquid Coconut Oil 1/2 cup peanut butter 1/2 cup cashew milk

Directions:

Take a saucepan, place it over medium heat, add all the ingredients except for oats and vanilla, stir until mixed, and then bring the mixture to boil. Simmer the mixture for 4 minutes, mixing frequently, then remove the pan from heat and stir in vanilla. Add oats, stir until well mixed and then scoop the mixture on a plate lined with wax paper. Serve straight away.

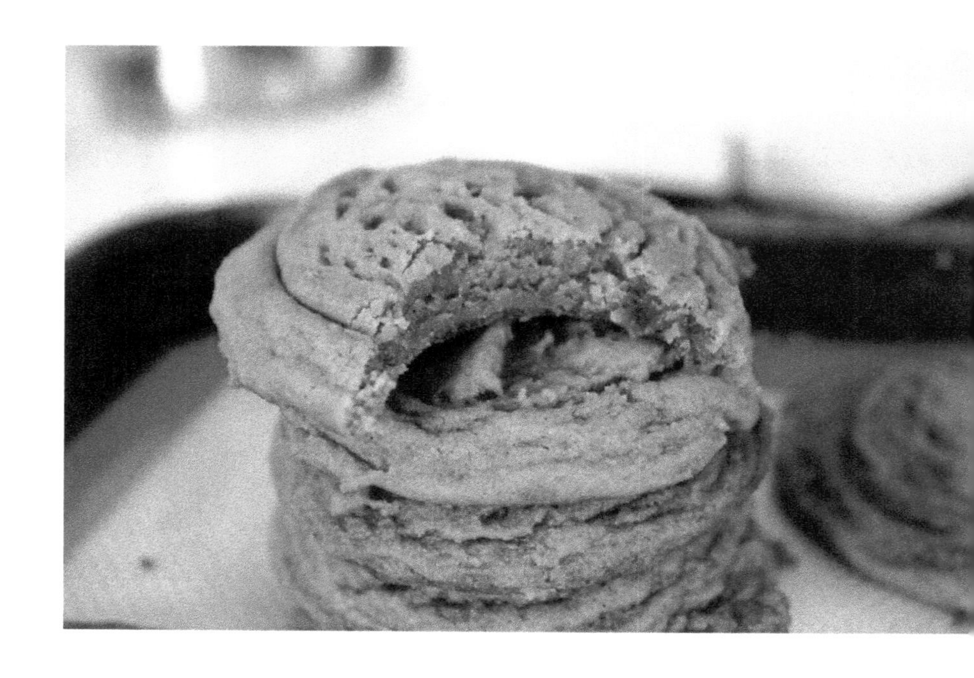

Mango Ice Cream

Preparation time: 5 minutes Cooking time: 0 minute Servings: 1

Ingredients:

2 frouncesen bananas, sliced 1 cup diced frouncesen mango

Directions:

Place all the ingredients in a food processor and pulse for 2 minutes until smooth. Distribute the ice cream mixture between two bowls and then serve immediately.

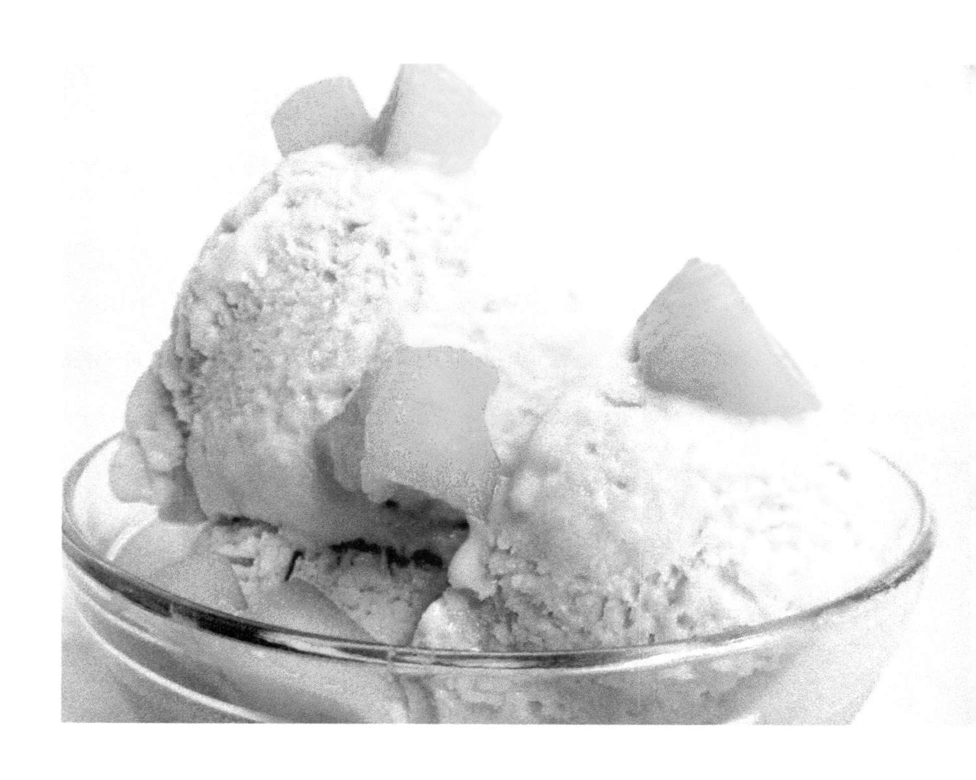

Blueberry Ice Cream

Preparation time: 5 minutes Cooking time: 0 minute Servings: 2

Ingredients:

2 frouncesen bananas, sliced ½ cup blueberries

Directions:

Place all the ingredients in a food processor and pulse for 2 minutes until smooth. Distribute the ice cream mixture between two bowls and then serve immediately.

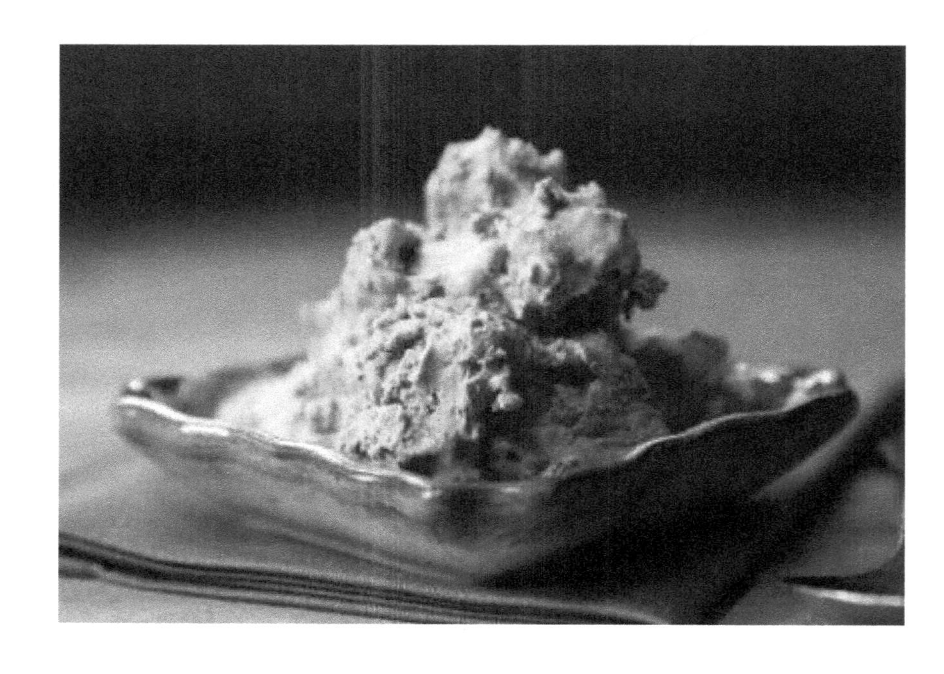

Whipped Cream

Preparation time: 5 minutes Cooking time: 0 minute Servings: 2

Ingredients:

¼ cup powdered sugar 1 teaspoon vanilla extract, unsweetened 14 ounces coconut milk, unsweetened, chilled

Directions:

Take a bowl, chill it overnight in the freezer, then separate coconut milk and solid and add solid from coconut milk into the chilled bowl. Add remaining ingredients and beat for 3 minutes until smooth and well combined. Serve straight away.

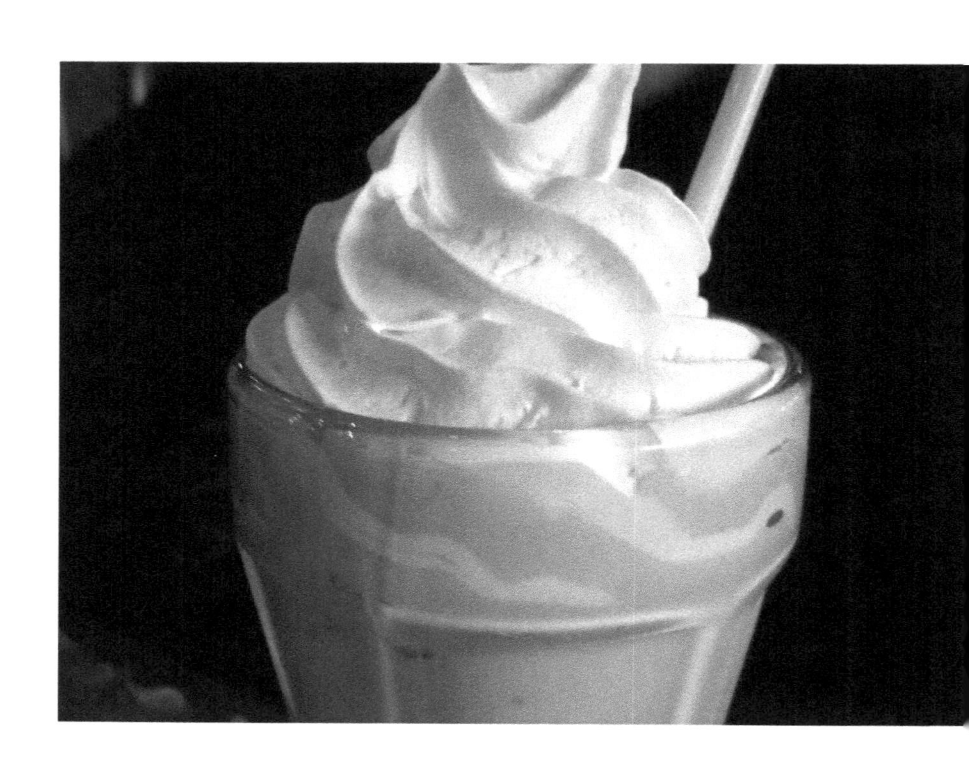

Peanut Butter Fudge

Preparation time: 50 minutes Cooking time: 1 minute Servings: 8

Ingredients:

1/2 cup peanut butter 2 tablespoons maple syrup 1/4 teaspoon salt 2 tablespoons coconut oil, melted 1/4 teaspoon vanilla extract, unsweetened

Directions:

Take a heatproof bowl, place all the ingredients in it, microwave for 15 seconds, and then stir until well combined. Take a freezer-proof container, line it with parchment paper, pour in fudge mixture, spread evenly and freeze for 40 minutes until set and harden. When ready to eat, let fudge set for 5 minutes, then cut it into squares and serve.

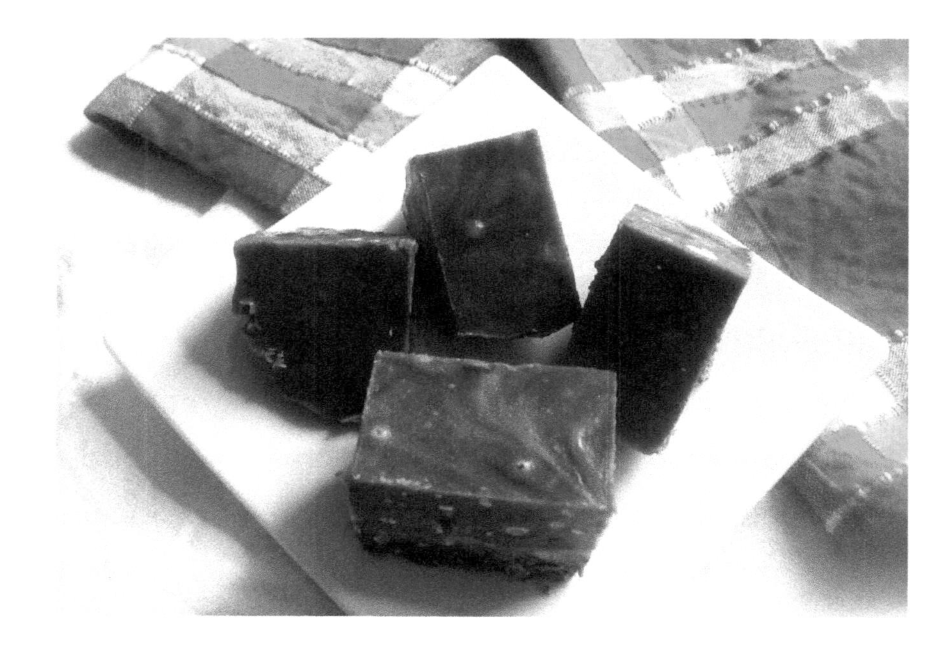

Gingerbread Energy Bites

Preparation time: 40 minutes Cooking time: 5 minutes Servings: 14

Ingredients:

12 dates, pitted, chopped 1 cup toasted pecans 2 ounces dark chocolate ¼ teaspoon cloves 1 teaspoon ground ginger 1 tablespoon molasses 1 teaspoon cinnamon ¼ teaspoon salt ¼ teaspoon ground nutmeg

Directions:

Place all the ingredients in a food processor, except for chocolate, pulse for 2 minutes until combined. Shape the mixture into 1-inch balls and place the balls on a cookie sheet lined with wax paper. Place chocolate in a heatproof bowl, microwave for 2 minutes until it has melted, stirring every 30 seconds. Pour the melted chocolate in a piping bag, drizzle it over prepared balls, refrigerate for 30 minutes until chocolate has hardened, and then serve.

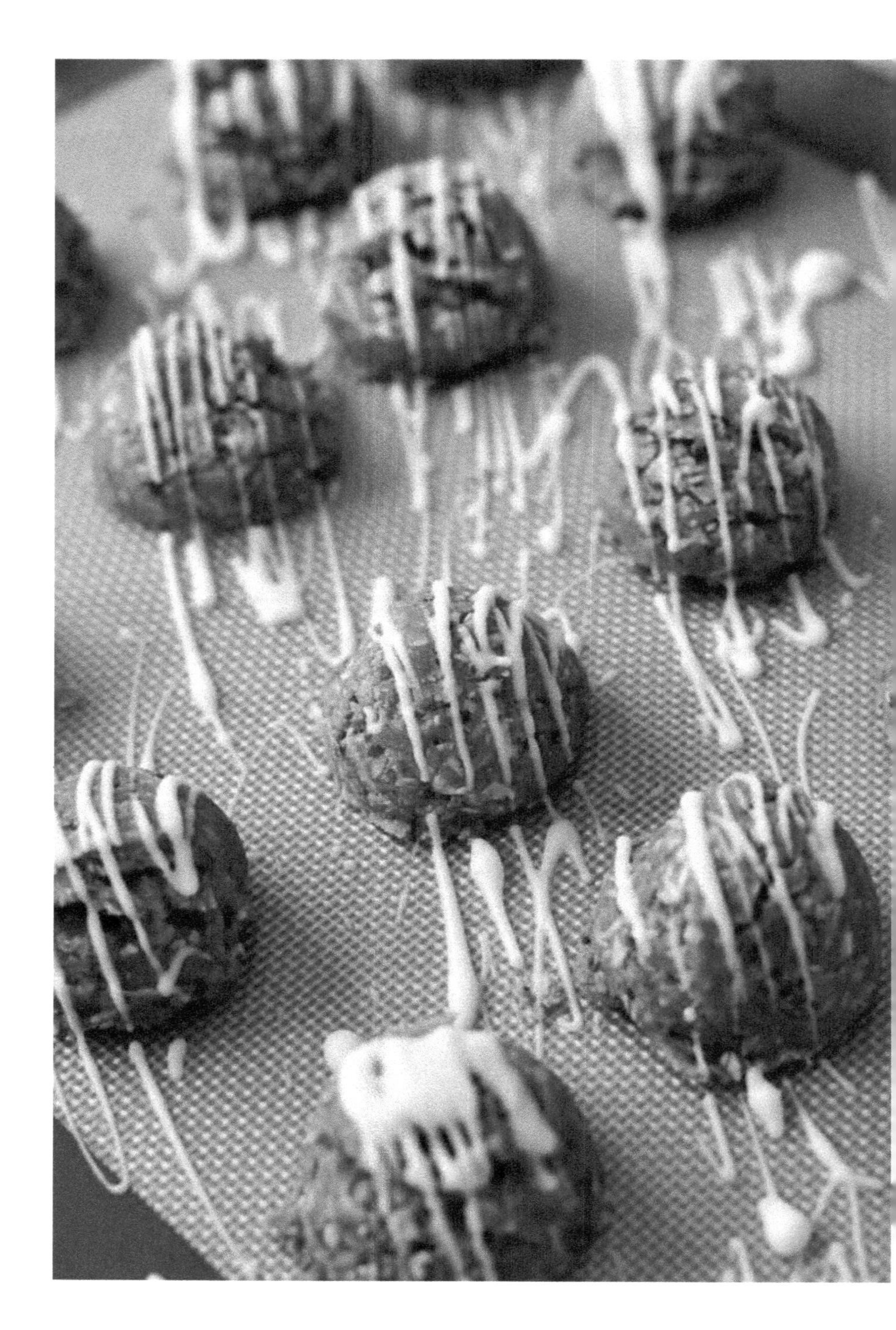

Peanut Butter Mousse

Preparation time: 50 minutes Cooking time: 0 minute Servings: 5

Ingredients:

3 Tablespoons agave nectar 14 ounces coconut milk, unsweetened, chilled 4 Tablespoons creamy peanut butter, salted

Directions:

Separate coconut milk and its solid, then add solid from coconut milk into the bowl and beat for 45 seconds until fluffy. Then beat in remaining ingredients until smooth, refrigerate for 45 minutes and serve.

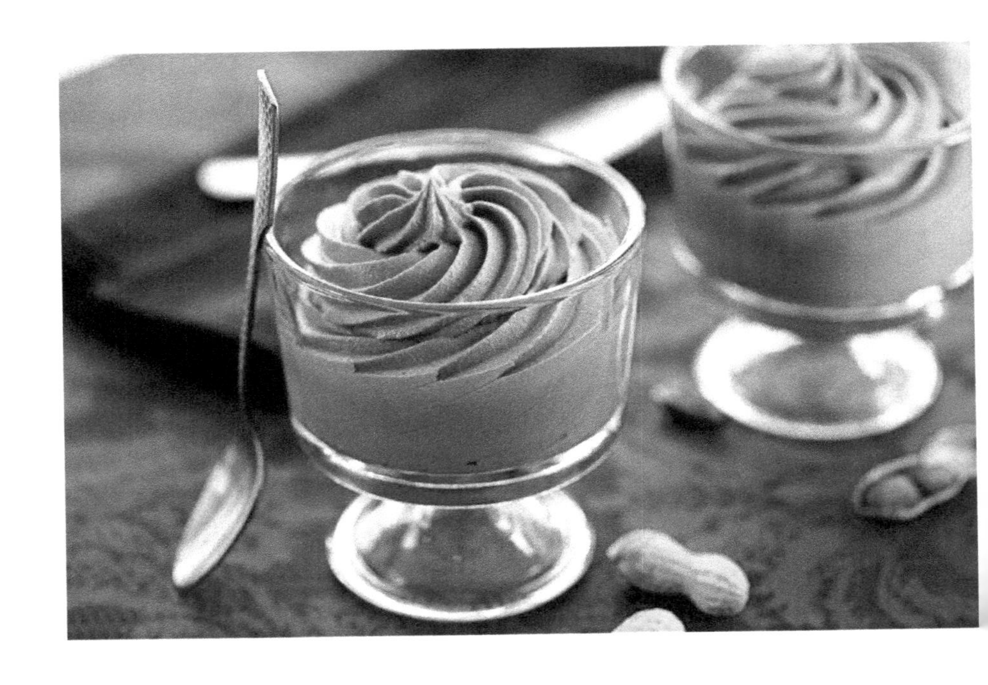

Mint Chocolate Chip Cheesecake

Preparation time: 5 hours and 15 minutes Cooking time 0 minuteServings: 6

Ingredients:

For the Crust: 7.5 ounces hazelnuts 2 tablespoons cocoa powder 3.5 ounces dates, pitted 1.5 ounces dark chocolate, melted 1/8 teaspoon salt 1 tablespoon coconut oil, melted

For the Mint Layer: ½ cup spinach leaves 7 ounces cashew nuts, soaked in warm water for 10 minutes 1/3 cup coconut oil, melted 1 teaspoon vanilla extract, unsweetened 1/4 cup maple syrup 3 teaspoons mint extract, unsweetened

Directions:

Prepare the crust, and for this, place all its ingredients in a food processor and pulse for 3 to 5 minutes until the thick paste comes together. Take a cake tin, line it with baking paper, pour crust mixture in it and spread and press the mixture evenly in the bottom, and freeze until required. Prepare mint layer and for this, drain cashews, transfer them into a food processor, add remaining ingredients, and pulse for 8 minutes until smooth. Pour the creamy mint mixture into prepared crust, smooth the top and freeze for 4 hours until set. Decorate the cake with mint leaves, cut it into slices, and then serve.

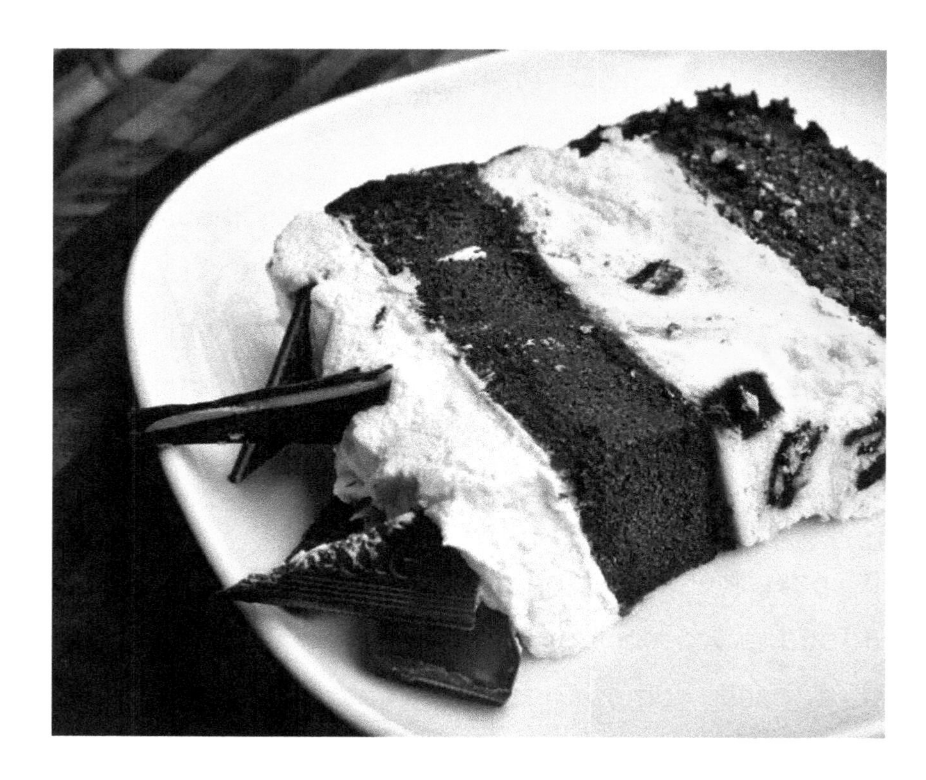

Coconut Lemon Tart

Preparation time: 3 hours and 15 minutes Cooking time: 10 minutes Servings: 8

Ingredients:

For the Crust: 1/2 cup shredded coconut, unsweetened 1/2 cup almonds 1/2 cup pecans 1/2 cup dates

For the Filling: 1/2 tablespoon lemon zest 2 tablespoons cornstarch 1/2 cup agave nectar 1 1/2 cups and 2 tablespoons lemon juice 1/2 teaspoon agar powder 7.5 ounces coconut cream 1/4 cup water

Directions:

Prepare the crust, and for this, place all its ingredients in a food processor and pulse for 3 to 5 minutes until the thick paste comes together. Take a 10-inch pie pan, dust it lightly with coconut, pour crust mixture in it and spread and press the mixture evenly in the bottom and sides, and freeze until required. Prepare the filling and for this, place a saucepan, place it over medium-low heat, add all the ingredients of filling, and whisk well and simmer for 10 minutes until the filling has thickened, whisking constantly. Let filling cool for 5 minutes, pour the filling into the prepared tart, smooth the top and freeze for 3 hours until set. Cut tart into slices and then serve.

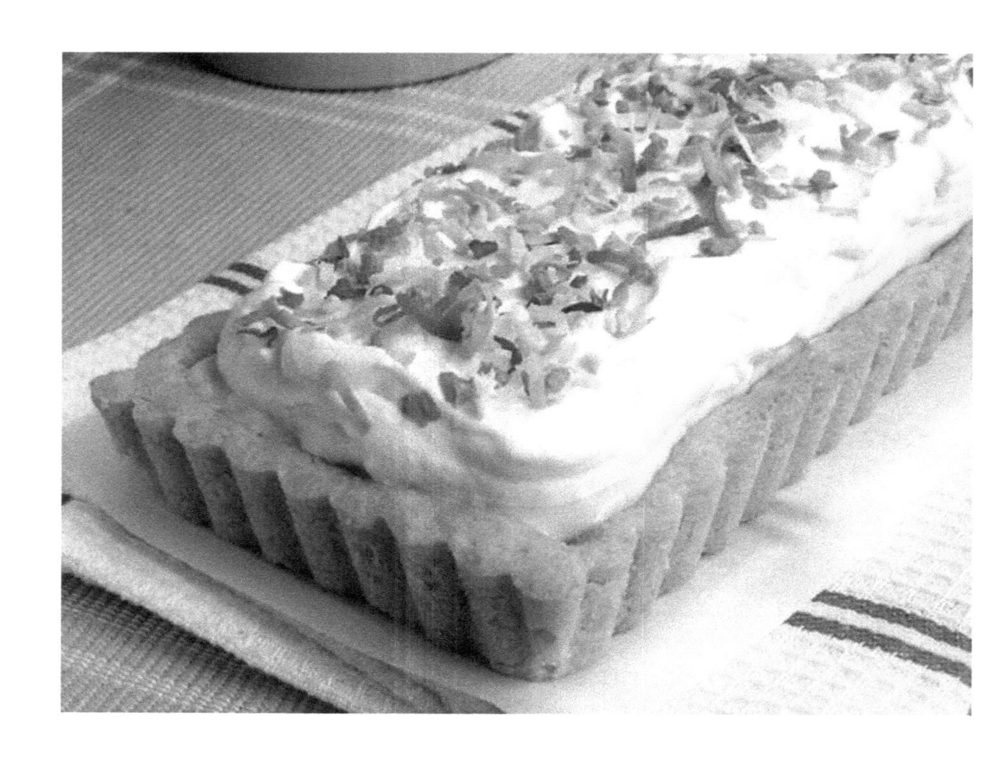

Chocolate Banana Cream Cake

Preparation time:6 hours and 15 minutes Cooking time:0 minute Servings: 4

Ingredients:

For the Crust:

2 tablespoons coconut cream 2 tablespoons coconut flour 1/8 teaspoon sea salt 1 1 tablespoon xylitol sweetener 1/8 teaspoon cinnamon 1 tablespoon almond butter

For the Banana Layer: 1 banana, sliced For the Chocolate Cream Layer: 1 tablespoon cacao powder 1/8 teaspoon sea salt 1/8 teaspoon cinnamon 1 tablespoon xylitol sweetener 4 tablespoons melted coconut oil 2 tablespoons coconut milk For the Coconut Whipped Cream: 1 tablespoon xylitol sweetener 14 ounces coconut cream, chilled

For Toppings: Cacao nibs as needed Cinnamon powder as needed

Directions:

Prepare the crust and for this, take a bowl, place all its ingredients in it and whisk until well combined. Take a small tin, line it with parchment paper, place crust mixture in it, spread and press the mixture evenly in the bottom, then layer with banana and freeze until required. Prepare the chocolate cream and for this, take a bowl, place all its ingredients in it and whisk until wel combined. Pour the chocolate cream over the banana layer in the prepared cake tin and return to the freezer until set. Then prepare the coconut whipped cream and for this, take a bowl, place cream in it, beat at high speed until thickened, and then beat in sugar until mixed. When cake has set, spread whipped cream on top, continue freezing until set and then slice to serve.

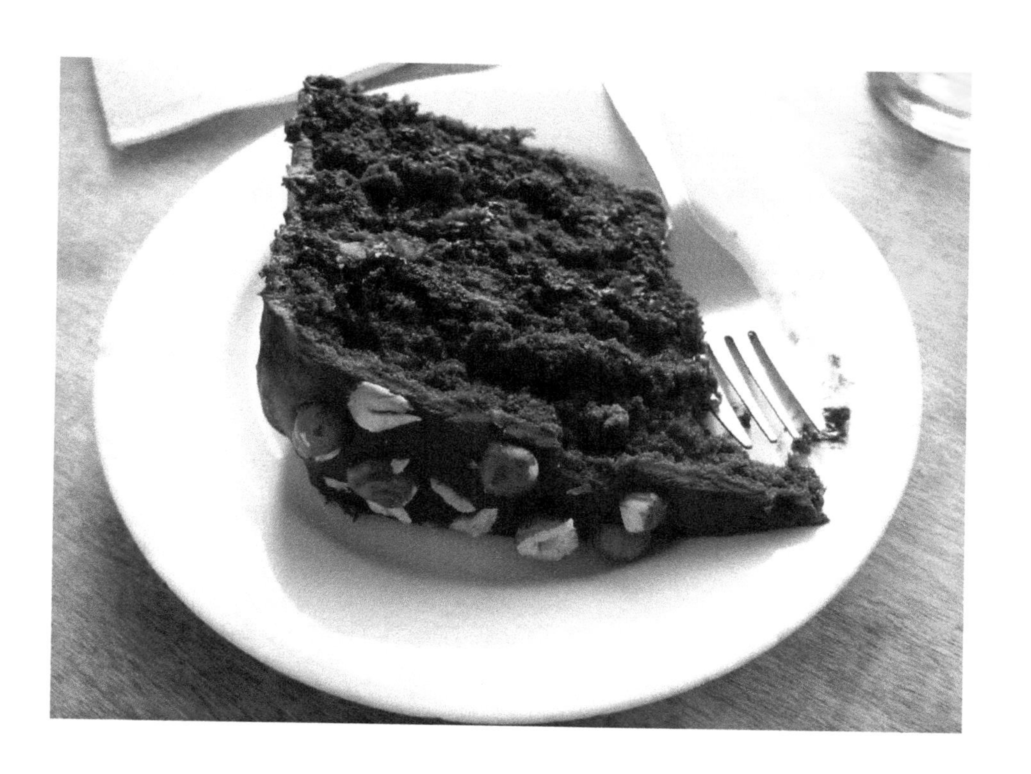

Key Lime Pie

Preparation time:3 hours and15 minutes Cooking time:0 minuteServings: 12

Ingredients:

For the Crust: ¾ cup coconut flakes, unsweetened 1 cup dates, soaked in warm water for 10 minutes in water, drained

For the Filling: ¾ cup of coconut meat 1 ½ avocado, peeled, pitted 2 tablespoons key lime juice ¼ cup agave

Directions:

Prepare the crust, and for this, place all its ingredients in a food processor and pulse for 3 to 5 minutes until the thick paste comes together. Take an 8-inch pie pan, grease it with oil, pour crust mixture in it and spread and press the mixture evenly in the bottom and along the sides, and freeze until required. Prepare the filling and for this, place all its ingredients in a food processor, and pulse for 2 minutes until smooth. Pour the filling into prepared pan, smooth the top, and freeze for 3 hours until set. Cut pie into slices and then serve.

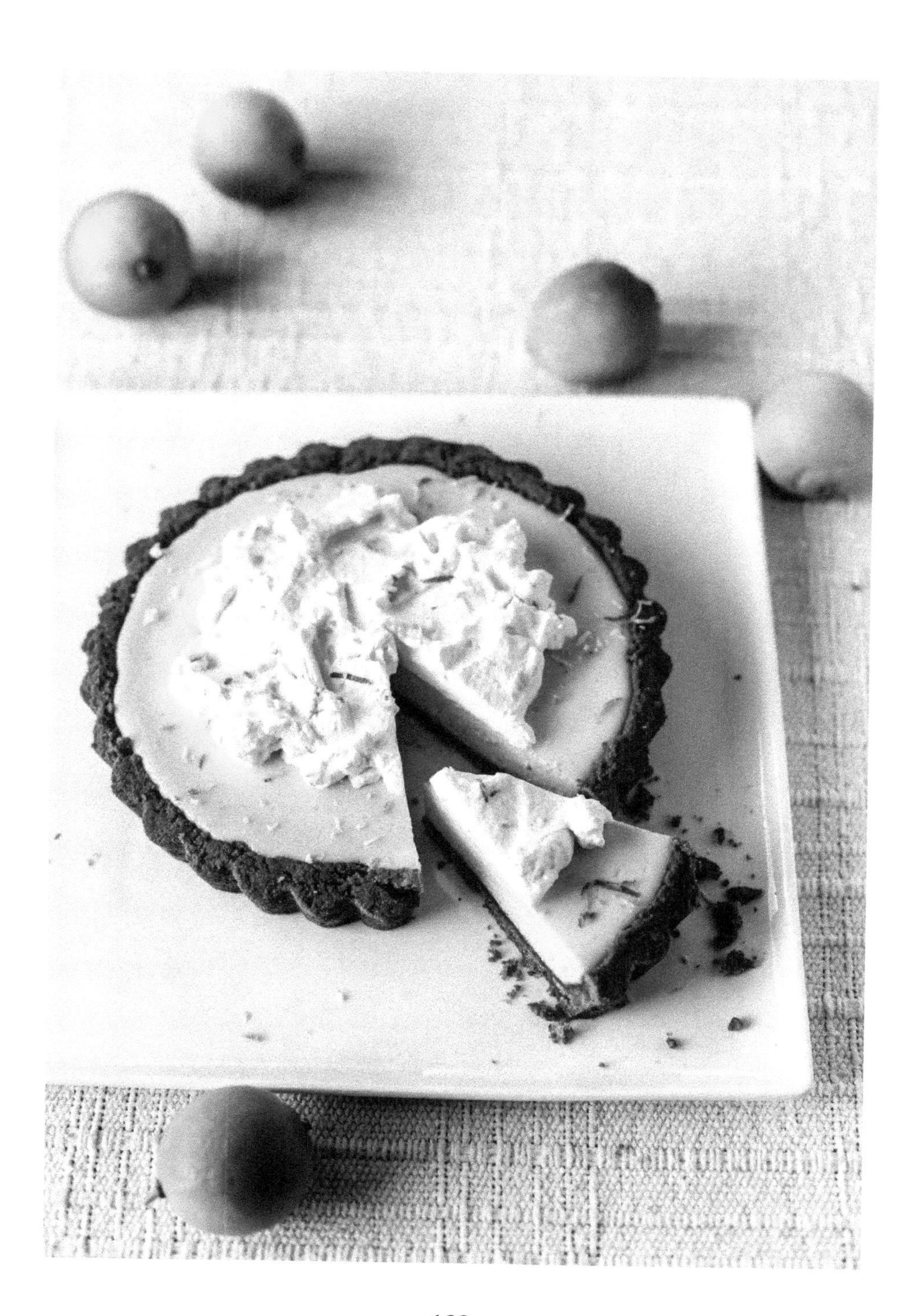

Lightning Source UK Ltd.
Milton Keynes UK
UKHW020700240521
384264UK00005B/100